COMPLETE GUIDE TO
NATURAL
HOME REMEDIES

COMPLETE GUIDE TO

NATURAL
HOME REMEDIES

Over 100 Recipes
Essential Oils, Herbs, and Natural Ingredients
to Treat Common Aches and Pains

Melissa Corkhill

IMM **lifestyle**
books™
Read. Learn. Do What You Love.

© 2024 by Melissa Corkhill and Fox Chapel Publishing Company, Inc., 903 Square Street, Mount Joy, PA 17552.

Portions of *Complete Guide to Natural Home Remedies* (2024) are taken from Self-Sufficiency: Natural Home Remedies (2016), published by IMM Lifestyle Books; an imprint of Fox Chapel Publishing Company, Inc.

ISBN 978-1-5048-0137-9

Library of Congress Control Number: 2023943858

The views expressed in this book are the author's own and do not necessarily represent those of Fox Chapel Publishing.

Disclaimer: This book should not be considered a replacement for professional medical treatment; a physician should be consulted on all matters relating to health. While the information in this book is believed to be accurate, the publisher cannot accept any legal responsibility for any injury or illness sustained while following given advice.

To learn more about the other great books from Fox Chapel Publishing, or to find a retailer near you, call toll-free 800-457-9112 or visit us at *www.FoxChapelPublishing.com*.

We are always looking for talented authors. To submit an idea, please send a brief inquiry to acquisitions@foxchapelpublishing.com.

Printed in China
First printing

CONTENTS

Getting Started. 8
   Introduction. 8
   How to Use This Book 11
   Plant Knowledge 12
   Essential Home Remedy Kit 13
   Your Herbal First Aid Kit. 15
   Growing Your Own Medicine. 18
   Creating an Herb Spiral 18

Treating Ailments. 25

Mind and Emotions 26
   Addiction 28
   Anxiety 29
   Memory Loss 29
   Depression 30
   Insomnia. 31
   Obsessive-Compulsive Disorder (OCD) . . . 32
   Phobias 33
   Stress 34
   Plant Profile: Rose. 37

Nervous System. 39
   Multiple Sclerosis 39
   Stroke 41
   Parkinson's Disease. 41
   Shingles. 42
   Migraine 43
   Headache 44
   Neuralgia 45
   Epilepsy. 45
   Plant Profile: Rosemary 46

Digestive System 48
  Nausea and Vomiting. 50
  Gastroenteritis 51
  Stomachache 51
  Travel Sickness. 51
  Indigestion and Heartburn 52
  Constipation 52
  Diarrhea 53
  Irritable Bowel Syndrome (IBS) 53
  Flatulence 54
  Hepatitis 54
  Crohn's Disease 55
  Plant Profile: Dandelion. *56*
  Plant Profile: Milk Thistle *59*

Urinary System 61
  Kidney Stones 62
  Urinary Complaints 63
  Cystitis 63
  Stress Incontinence. 63
  Urine Therapy 64
  Plant Profile: Nettle *65*

Respiratory System 67
  Flu 68
  Hay Fever 69
  Common Cold. 70

Sinusitis 71
Nosebleeds 72
Sore Throat. 72
Cough 73
Asthma 73
Pneumonia. 73
Lung Infection/Bronchitis 74
Catarrh 75
Plant Profile: Lavender. *76*

The Skin 79
  Eczema 81
  Psoriasis 82
  Prickly Heat 82
  Perspiration 83
  Acne. 84
  Athlete's Foot 85
  Chilblains 85
  Cuts and Sores 86
  Cold Sores. 87
  Sunstroke 87
  Rashes 88
  Warts. 88
  Boils. 89
  Hair Loss. 89
  Dandruff. 90
  Sunburn 90
  Insect Bites 91
  Plant Profile: Calendula. *92*

Heart and Blood Health 94
  High Blood Pressure 97
  Low Blood Pressure 97
  Anemia 98
  Angina. 98
  Hemorrhoids 99
  Varicose Veins 100
  Plant Profile: Hawthorn. *101*

Bones, Muscles, and Joints. 103
  Osteoporosis 104
  Sprains and Pulled Muscles. 105

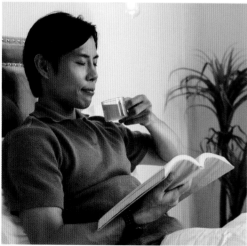

Fractures. 105

Rheumatism. 106

Backache. 107

Arthritis. 108

Plant Profile: Comfrey 110

Eyes and Ears. 112

Conjunctivitis 114

Eyestrain. 115

Styes 116

Ear Wax Buildup. 116

Middle Ear Infection. 117

Plant Profile: Fennel. 118

Women's Health 121

Menstrual Cycle. 123

Fertility 125

Pregnancy. 126

Pregnancy Anemia 127

Pregnancy Backache 127

Pregnancy Constipation. 128

Bleeding Gums 128

Cramps 129

Pregnancy Indigestion 129

Pregnancy Insomnia. 130

Fluid Retention 130

Dizziness. 130

Morning Sickness 130

Pelvic Pain 131

Pregnancy Hemorrhoids 131

Stretch Marks. 131

Thrush. 132

Tiredness 133

Childbirth. 134

Breastfeeding. 135

Milk Production 136

Sore, Cracked Nipples 136

Engorgement 137

Problems with Let-Down. 138

Inflammation. 139

Fatigue. 139

Menopause. 140

Plant Profile: Motherwort 142

Plant Profile: Sweet Violet 144

Babies and Children 146

Sore Throat and Coughs. 147

Colds. 148

Croup 148

Chicken pox 148

Earache 149

Eczema 149

Head Lice 150

Measles 151

Diaper Rash 151

Teething 151

Fever 152

Mumps 153

Plant Profile: Chamomile. 154

Index. 156

Photo Credits. 159

About the Author 160

GETTING STARTED

Nature provides us with a wealth of natural remedies that can help to ease and soothe illnesses, ailments, and common health complaints. The following pages contain all you need to know to begin treating yourself and your family by increasing your plant knowledge, putting together an herbal first aid kit, and even growing your own medicine.

Introduction

I started this journey as a child, always fascinated by plants and intrigued at the natural remedies that my mother used to treat us when my brother, sister, and I were ill. She had a huge collection of homeopathic remedies and through her treating us, I learned about many of them, what they were made from, and what symptoms they could be used to treat. I came to understand that a heavy cold

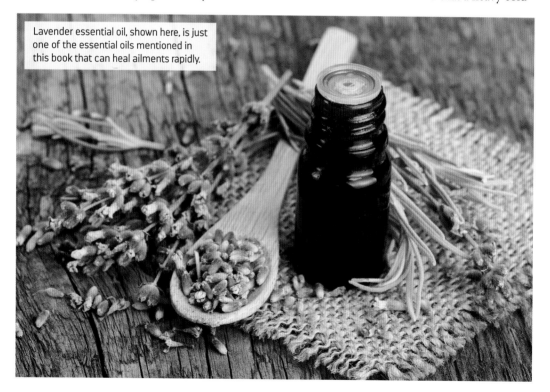

Lavender essential oil, shown here, is just one of the essential oils mentioned in this book that can heal ailments rapidly.

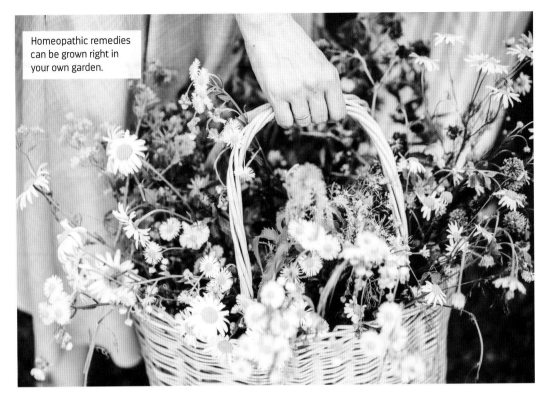

Homeopathic remedies can be grown right in your own garden.

could benefit from a dose of Pulsatilla, that a case of nerves before an exam was effectively treated using Gelsemium, and that a hot honey and lemon drink was the best remedy for a sore throat.

When my own children were born, I started to use natural remedies to treat their illnesses. Eventually, as they got older, they were able to decide what remedy would work best for them. They now instinctively know what plant will be most effective to help their bodies to heal. I have learned to trust their innate knowledge, and at the time of writing none of us has seen a doctor in seventeen years! We are our own doctors, which is a liberating feeling.

No one can know and understand your body better than you can. I like to do a body scan meditation occasionally, to give my body a chance to really let me know how it is feeling and to identify any problem areas that need attention. To do this, simply lie down in a comfortable place where you can be sure that you won't be disturbed for at least twenty minutes. Bring your attention to your feet. Think about how they feel. Give your body time to respond, as you may not be used to focusing on individual parts in this way. If you can't decide how your feet are feeling the first time, don't worry, simply move to your ankles and focus on them.

Slowly move up your body, thinking about how it is feeling, until you get to the head. You may have thoughts such as, "I'm tired; I feel confused; I feel stuck." After you have worked through

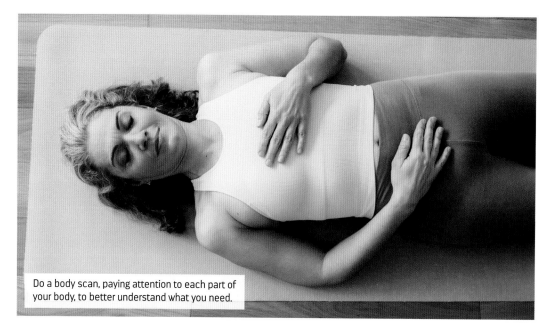

Do a body scan, paying attention to each part of your body, to better understand what you need.

the whole body, sit up and jot down each of the messages from your body parts so that you have a reference to work with over the coming weeks. You can then refer to the advice given in this book to treat and heal any problem areas.

When parts of my body feel stiff or blocked, I use yoga and herbs to help me release the tension. Yoga is an incredible therapy for moving and releasing blockages that might go on to cause illness if allowed to build up. For example, I developed a benign lump in my breast thirteen years ago, and through the practice of yoga and use of natural remedies I managed to shift the blockage and now feel healthier than ever.

In this book, I will share remedies and techniques that I have used myself for decades and on my children for over twenty years. Many of the recipes for healing lotions, infusions, and tinctures are ones that we use regularly in our home. I hope that they will be useful for you to help you create optimum health for you and your family.

A hot honey and lemon drink, like this one, heals a sore throat.

How to Use This Book

I have divided this book up into bodily systems, so you will find remedies for the respiratory system in one chapter and how to heal disorders of the digestive system in another (see the illustration below). I prefer to work with the body as a whole rather than just the symptoms, but for ease of use and understanding I have chosen to organize the book in this way. You may find that you need to look in more than one section to find a selection of treatments that work for you. For example, if your child has chicken pox, you'll find some useful remedies

You will learn how to use the plants in your garden, like comfrey here, into healing salves.

in the Babies and Children section on page 146. However, you may also want to check out the Skin chapter on page 79 to find ways to help soothe the inflamed rash that accompanies the chicken pox virus. Alongside the remedies are plenty of recipes that you can create at home.

This book is designed to empower you to be able to take control of your own health using your kitchen and garden. You will also find instructions on how to create a healing herb garden and in each chapter a spotlight on one of my favorite herbal healers. I have chosen plants that are well known, easy to find, and that I use regularly at home, such as nettles, rose, lavender, and comfrey. In addition, I have put together my suggestions for an herbal first aid kit (see page 15) that you can have on hand for emergencies, including my top recommendations for treatments to carry when out and about.

Bodily Systems

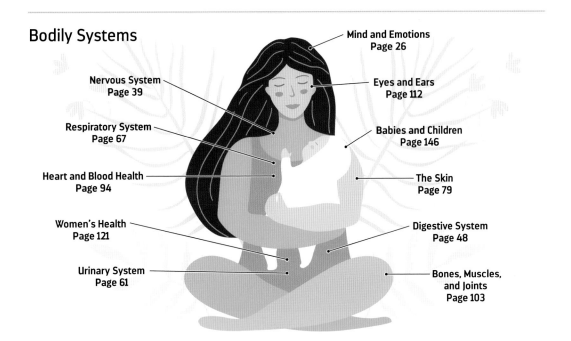

Mind and Emotions
Page 26

Nervous System
Page 39

Eyes and Ears
Page 112

Respiratory System
Page 67

Babies and Children
Page 146

Heart and Blood Health
Page 94

The Skin
Page 79

Women's Health
Page 121

Digestive System
Page 48

Urinary System
Page 61

Bones, Muscles, and Joints
Page 103

Plant Knowledge

It is a good idea to familiarize yourself with what plants grow in your area. Spend time in the garden with a notebook to record what you find. Make drawings, press leaves and flowers between the pages, and take notes. It doesn't have to be scientific. Write down what you see and how you interpret the plants around you. Ask questions—does it have large or small leaves? What are they shaped like? Is it flowering now? Where is the plant growing—in shade or full sun? Soon you will start to build up a good knowledge of the plants growing in your backyard, then you can start to learn about their healing properties. Don't expect this knowledge

Take a notebook and record what you find in your garden or around your neighborhood.

to come all at once. I have been working with and learning about plants for over twenty-five years and there is still so much more to learn, but each season I gather a bit more knowledge about what I can use to help heal my family.

Once you have studied the plants in your area, take your notebook further afield and observe the hedgerows around your home, local wasteland, or park. Make notes on what is growing or flowering now, what is coming up, and where you found it. Highlight plants to visit again in a couple of weeks' time. For example, if you spot an elder covered with tiny white buds in mid spring, make a note to come back in a week and you'll be rewarded with plumes of frothy white flowers that can be harvested to make an excellent remedy for hay fever. Soon, you will have built up knowledge of your local plants; you will possess an invaluable resource for when it comes to treating your body holistically.

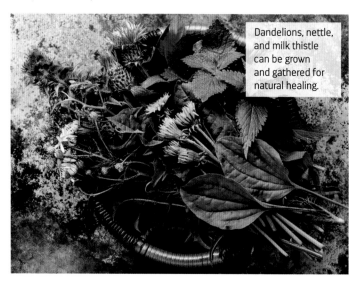

Dandelions, nettle, and milk thistle can be grown and gathered for natural healing.

You can use your knowledge to create a map of natural healing remedies that are easily accessible in your area. It will soon start to become second nature to brew up a batch of nettle tonic in early spring or to harvest a couple of handfuls of hawthorn berries in the autumn to make a hearty concoction of hawthorn brandy that can be used to treat heart conditions in the months ahead.

Essential Home Remedy Kit

To learn about natural remedies, it is a good idea to build up a toolkit of home medicines that you can try out on yourself, your family, and friends. I have listed some of the basic remedies that I like to have on hand here.

It is helpful to have the remedies that you use frequently on hand, so that they are easily accessible when you need them. I have a shelf in a kitchen cupboard where I keep some of my remedies. Others, such as garlic, can be found in the vegetable basket or as herbs, growing in pots by the front door. You might like to include a notebook in your kit. This can be useful for noting down what you have used, on what date, on whom you used it, and how effective it was at treating the problem. This will be a great source of information for your family when a similar problem occurs.

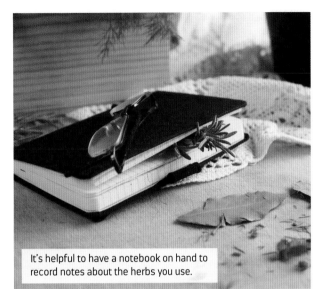

It's helpful to have a notebook on hand to record notes about the herbs you use.

Toolkit Basics

Garlic

A powerful treatment for a range of ailments. Use raw as a decongestant and to treat infection. I like to make it into a syrup with honey for chesty coughs and colds.

Lemon Juice

Has antibacterial qualities and is very cleansing. Combined with honey, lemon juice makes a soothing treatment for colds and coughs.

Aloe Vera

I have several pots of this succulent growing around the house. It can be used on burns, stings, and irritated skin to give almost instant relief.

Cloves

Excellent for treating toothache as they act as an analgesic. Pop one in your mouth and chew on it until the pain subsides.

Honey

An effective treatment for burns, it can also be used to make a soothing drink for sore throats and colds.

Lavender oil

I like to always have a supply of this essential oil available. It can be used on bites and stings, cuts, and wounds to help the skin to heal and applied to the temples to soothe a headache.

Calendula

I keep this on hand as an ointment to treat sore, irritated skin and just to use as a lip balm or moisturizer. I like to grow it in the herb beds for the beautiful sunshiny flowers, which can be used in several skincare preparations and as a colorful addition to a salad.

Peppermint

Peppermint tea can be used to treat indigestion or headaches. Pick a handful and steep in boiling water for ten minutes. Strain and drink as it is, or sweeten with honey to taste.

Ginger

Grated into boiling water to make a tea, this root will soothe respiratory and digestive problems. Combine with lemon juice and honey to make a powerful remedy for colds and coughs.

Chamomile

Whenever anyone in my family gets an eye infection, I turn to chamomile tea. I've even used it on our pet guinea pigs and cat. Allow the tea to cool and bathe the infected eye using organic cotton pads or a clean flannel.

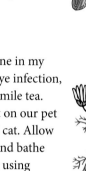

Comfrey

An ointment made from this plant is useful for treating bruises and bites. I have a large pot of this magical plant growing by the front door.

Arnica

I use the homeopathic remedy and cream regularly so always have some available at home. It can be used in cases of (non-medical) shock and to treat bumps and bruises.

Rescue remedy

Every home should have a little bottle of this blend of five flower essences. It can be used to treat mild shock, trauma, and injury. Take five drops on the tongue or dilute in a glass of water for younger children.

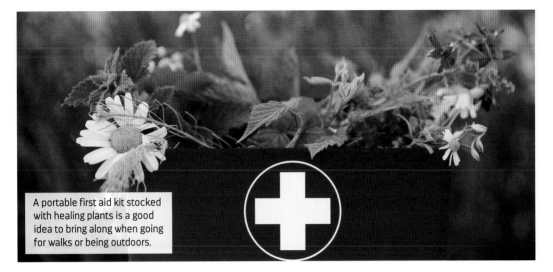

A portable first aid kit stocked with healing plants is a good idea to bring along when going for walks or being outdoors.

Your Herbal First Aid Kit

It is a good idea to put together a pack of remedies that can be used for first aid at home. There are many natural treatments that can easily be administered to treat the body in times of shock and distress. As well as having a good selection of remedies at home to treat emergencies, it might be worthwhile enrolling in a first aid course where you can learn the basics of administering first aid, such as how to deal with broken limbs and resuscitation skills before medical help arrives.

When putting together your natural first aid kit, you will want to have items such as bandages and a small pair of scissors as well as medicines made from plants. You may want to make up a smaller kit for taking out and about. A portable kit that fits easily in a backpack is a good idea for vacations, walks, and days out. Items that I would recommend for your portable first aid kit are marked with an asterisk. * = **recommended for your portable first aid kit**

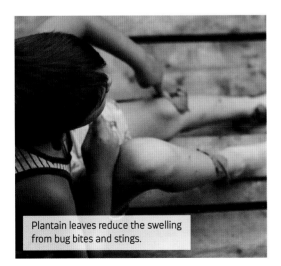

Plantain leaves reduce the swelling from bug bites and stings.

Bites and Stings

Stings are common and easily dealt with using natural remedies. If an allergic reaction occurs, seek the advice of a doctor.

Plantain can ease the pain and reduce swelling. Chew the leaf in your mouth and apply the masticated leaves as a poultice to the sting.

Lavender oil* can be applied directly to a sting.

Rescue remedy*. If the person who has been stung is in distress, five drops taken on the tongue will work to calm the patient.

Aloe vera can be applied to the affected area. Split a leaf and spread the juice onto the skin.

Mild shock

Mild shock can be successfully treated with natural remedies; however, this condition should not be confused with medical shock which always requires medical attention.

Rescue remedy* to treat a patient who has experienced trauma.

Chamomile tea can be calming for the nervous system. Brew a cup and encourage the patient to take small sips while still warm.

Lavender oil* can be used to alleviate shock. Place a few drops onto a handkerchief and inhale until the shock subsides.

Aconite, Arnica,* and **Ignatia** are all homeopathic remedies that can be used to treat shock and distress.

Apply the juice of aloe vera to the skin to ease the affected area.

Cuts and Wounds

If possible, raise the cut above the level of the heart (e.g. if the cut is on the arm, lift the arm above the head). Apply direct pressure to the area and continue until the flow of blood stops, or in more serious cases, until medical help arrives.

Aloe vera can be applied to cuts and grazes and will help skin to heal and prevent infection.

Tea tree* **or lavender oil*** are used to clean wounds with a few drops of each diluted in warm water. This will also act as an antiseptic.

Hypericum and **arnica*** are homeopathic remedies that can be used to help the body to heal.

Rescue remedy* can be applied directly to a graze to promote healing.

Comfrey ointment* can be applied to inflamed cuts. (See recipe below)

Comfrey Ointment

- 1¼ pounds (500 grams) soft beeswax
- 2¼ ounces (60 grams) dried (or 5 ounces / 150 grams fresh) comfrey leaves, finely chopped

1. Melt the beeswax in a glass bowl over a pan of boiling water.

2. Add the comfrey leaves and simmer, stirring continuously, for about 1 hour.

3. Pour the mixture into a muslin bag. Wearing rubber gloves, squeeze the mixture through the bag into a jug.

4. Pour the ointment into a jar before it sets. Place the lid on the jar without securing it.

5. When cool, tighten the lid and store in a refrigerator for up to 3 months.

Sunstroke

This is a type of heat exhaustion resulting from prolonged exposure to sun, often accompanied by headache, shivering, nausea, and dizziness.

Rescue remedy* will help the patient to recover. Take five drops in a glass of water and sip slowly.

Apply honey to the burn for a speedy recovery.

Burns and Scalds

First, pour cold liquid onto the burn or scald for at least ten minutes, then use whichever of the following treatments you have available.

Aloe vera will cool the area and prevent infection. Split a leaf and gently apply the juice to the affected area.

Honey will help the skin to heal. Apply to the affected area.

Lavender oil* can be used neat on a burn to promote healing and prevent infection. Gently massage a few drops into the affected area.

Sipping chamomile tea can soothe the digestive system.

Food Poisoning

Warm water mixed with the juice of half a lemon will help to cleanse the system.

Honey can be dissolved in a glass of warm water and sipped frequently to increase strength and boost the immune system.

Bio live yogurt can be eaten after the vomiting has subsided to help repopulate the stomach with beneficial bacteria.

Chamomile tea can be calming and soothing for the digestive system. A tonic can be made using herbs from the kitchen cupboard, which will help to cleanse the system.

Cleansing Tonic

- 1 teaspoon black pepper
- 2 cloves garlic, crushed
- 1 tablespoon cumin seeds
- Pinch of salt
- 1 pint (600 ml) water

1. Place ingredients into a pan and boil until the liquid is reduced by half.

2. Drink twice a day to help cleanse the system and to treat diarrhea.

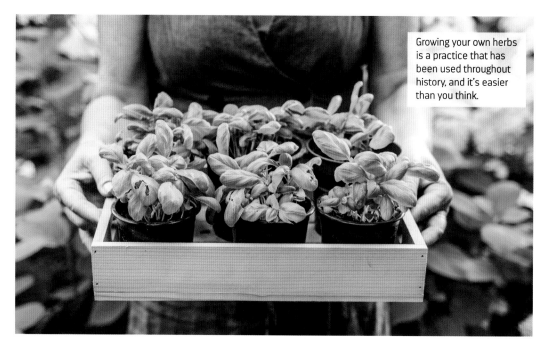

Growing your own herbs is a practice that has been used throughout history, and it's easier than you think.

Growing Your Own Medicine

Herbs have been used throughout history as medicines, perfumes, insect repellents, and of course, in food. In most cases, herbs are perennial and are tough wild plants which, when introduced to the luxurious conditions of a garden, will thrive. Planting your own medicine garden is a simple, pleasurable activity that will benefit you and your family for many years to come. It is a good idea to plant a small herb garden near the house that you can use as a medicine chest. Apothecary gardens have been grown for centuries full of the healing powers of plants.

Positioning your herb bed as close to the house as possible will make tending and harvesting easier. When planning an apothecary garden remember that not all herbs like full sun; divide the area into sun, partial shade, and full shade and plant accordingly. I recommend selecting a circular plot and making an herb spiral.

Creating an Herb Spiral

An herb spiral is as simple as it sounds: a large spiral structure, typically measuring 1½–2 yards/meters-wide diameter at the base, spiraling up to a height of around 1 yard, with a planting path running up it. An herb spiral of these proportions is big enough to accommodate at least all the basic herbs included here, and a few slightly more exotic ones, too.

There are many advantages of creating an herb spiral. First, by making use of both the vertical and the horizontal space, it allows you to make maximum use of a small growing area. This is particularly beneficial to those with little or no garden. The curved nature of the planting beds also increases the growing area available, compared to more traditional straight-edged gardens. Due to its design, the herb spiral offers a variety of different microclimates and aspects that are all easily accessible.

The benefits of this diversity of habitats are obvious—the gardener can plant a wide range of plants, all with differing needs and uses, in a very small area. Oil-rich herbs, such as rosemary, thyme, and sage can be grown on the dry and sunny top-southerly side, whereas the moist and sheltered base on the northerly side is perfect for green foliage herbs such as mint, parsley, and coriander. There is even the potential to create a small pond or bog area at the base of the spiral for plants such as watercress and water mint.

Virtually any building materials can be used to construct the herb spiral, as long as they're reasonably long-lived and not likely to rot away as untreated wood is liable to do. Anything from wooden stakes to large slates, bricks, stones, bottles stacked on their side, or even scrap tires can be used to create the walls of the spiral. If you are building directly onto earth, it's advisable to mulch the area beforehand, to prevent weed problems while the herbs are establishing themselves. You can use anything water permeable, such as cardboard or old carpet. If you are building onto concrete, break it up to ensure adequate drainage.

You can choose one of two methods of construction. The simplest and possibly less-stable method, at least while the herbs are becoming established, is to pile the soil into a large heap and insert stones, slates, etc. to create a spiral shape. Because there is a danger of the soil washing away in rain or blowing away in wind before the plants are established, it is best to use pot-grown plants if you choose this method.

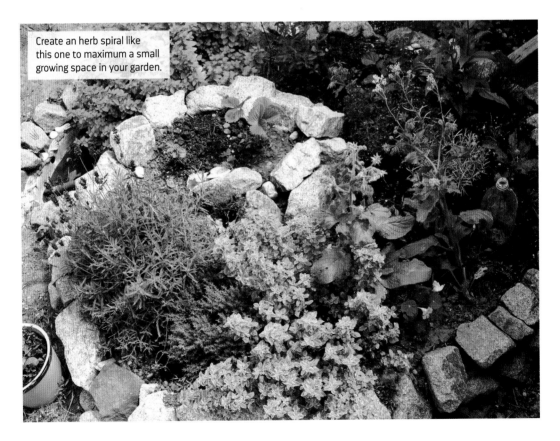

Create an herb spiral like this one to maximum a small growing space in your garden.

Once you construct your herb spiral, it will be easy to access all your herbs and vegetables.

The second method is more permanent and more involved. First, stake out the spiral shape using sticks or bamboo. The base should be between 1½–2 yards/meters in diameter. Next, construct the walls using bricks or stones, starting from the outside and moving inwards. Add more layers, gradually increasing the height as you move into the center. If you are using bricks and mortar, add the soil at the end. If you are using a "dry stone" technique (just stacking the stones on top of one another), add the soil as you go to give more support and stability.

Herbs for Your Herb Spiral

CALENDULA

This sunny annual has beautiful yellow-orange flowers that bloom from mid spring to early summer. It is one of the most widely used and effective medicinal plants. The flowers are loaded with healing properties including essential oils, saponins, carotenoid, and flavonoids. It can be used to heal wounds, reduce inflammations, and treat bruises, burns, and cuts. In skincare, it is used to treat acne, eczema, rosacea, and irritated or inflamed skin.

Grow: Sow seeds under cover in early spring—germination takes five to fourteen days—or sow direct into soil on the southern side of the herb spiral in late spring when risk of frost has passed.

Harvest: Pick flowers as soon as they open in early summer. Young leaves can be eaten in salads.

Uses: Good for diaper rash and skin complaints including cuts, grazes, minor burns, wounds, and fungal conditions. Sap from the stem has traditionally been used to treat warts, corns, and calluses.

LAVENDER

A woody perennial shrub with purple/bluish flowers that grow upwards on tall stems. It originated in the Mediterranean but now grows all over Europe and North America. The list of healing benefits of the lavender plant seems never-ending—it is anti-inflammatory, antispasmodic, and antiseptic. Essential oil can be applied direct to the skin to treat burns, bruising, and aching or tense muscles. In skincare the oil can be used to alleviate dry skin conditions, acne, dermatitis, and rosacea. It stimulates cell renewal and healing so is a useful ingredient in many skincare preparations.

Grow: Sow seeds under cover in spring. Germination takes around three weeks. Take softwood cuttings in late spring. Once these take root they can be planted up on the drier, southern side of the herb spiral.

Harvest: Cut flowers in summer just as they open.

Uses: Make a scented oil that can be used to relax and soothe tired bodies and minds. Place sachets of dried lavender leaves and flowers in wardrobes to deter moths or under pillows to aid sleep.

ROSEMARY

A hardy perennial evergreen with flower spikes of tiny violet blooms starting in early spring to early summer. Needle-shaped green leaves.

Grow: Sow under protection in early spring—germination takes seven to fourteen days—or take cuttings of new growth in summer after flowers have finished. Pot-up when well rooted and plant out on the southern banks of the herb spiral the following year.

Harvest: Pick leaves throughout the year.

Uses: As well as aiding memory retention and recovery from long-term illness, this herb can make a good insect repellent. Rub leaves into temples to alleviate headaches. A hair rinse can be made from the leaves.

CHAMOMILE

This hardy evergreen perennial produces large single white daisylike flowers throughout the summer. Leaves are green and sweet-smelling.

Grow: Start off in early spring under cover. Germination usually takes two to three weeks. Take cuttings or divide plants in the spring, to start new plants. They can then be planted-up on the eastern side of the herb spiral to catch the early-morning sun.

Harvest: Pick flowers as they open and dry them or use fresh.

Uses: Due to the plant's sedative properties the dried flowers are used to treat insomnia, digestive disorders, and travel sickness. A hair rinse can be made for fair hair. Tea made from the dried flowers can also be used to make a rinse for use in homemade baby wipes and as a treatment for irritated skin.

BORAGE

A pretty flowering hardy annual that originates from the Mediterranean. Also known as starflower, this herb was traditionally given to Roman soldiers for courage and comfort. The plant has several culinary and medicinal uses. Blue star-shaped flowers bloom from early summer to the first frosts. The mild-green leaves are bristly, oval, and succulent.

Grow: Sow seeds into pots in early spring under protection. Germination takes from five to fourteen days. When ready to plant out, position on the western side of the slopes of the herb spiral.

Harvest: Pick fresh flowers just as they begin to open fully. You can preserve them in ice cubes. The leaves taste good in soups and salads.

Uses: A facial steam for dry sensitive skin can be made with borage leaves as well as the flowers.

WILD STRAWBERRY

A hardy perennial with small white flowers that give way to tiny red fruit in the summer months. Leaves are also edible.

Grow: Pick fruit, dry them on cloth, and then rub off seeds into a tray of moist compost in the autumn. Germination takes six to ten weeks. Cover with a plastic bag to protect and keep warm. Plant out on the western side of the spiral when large enough to handle. The mature plants produce runners that can be trained into pots to make new plants. Place a pot full of compost under the green shoot at the end of the runner. Cut away from the main plant once rooted.

Harvest: Pick ripe fruit from summer through to early autumn.

Uses: Can be made into a treatment to prevent discoloration of the teeth.

OTHER POSSIBILITIES

Sweet violet: This creeping evergreen perennial grows to approximately 6 inches (15 cm). Both the leaves and flowers are tasty in winter salads. It can be used as a gentle expectorant and is excellent for breast health. Can be made into a poultice to treat breast lumps and mastitis.

Sorrel: This native perennial will reach a mature size of 24 inches (60 cm) high and 11¾ inches (30 cm) wide. It is very tolerant of a range of conditions, and is easily grown. Delicious when eaten in salads and a good source of nutrients.

Lemon balm: At maturity, this herb is 27½ inches (70 cm) tall and 16 inches (40 cm) wide. It is very tolerant of a range of conditions and will succeed in light shade. The lemon-flavored leaves can be used to make a refreshing tea that is uplifting and often used in treatment of depression or anxiety.

Wild garlic: Grows well in wet soils and will reach a height of up to 11¾ inches (30 cm). The garlic-flavored leaves are available in late winter/early spring and can be used in place of garlic in cooking.

TREATING AILMENTS

The following pages include many common ailments, illnesses, and medical conditions that can be successfully treated or soothed using natural remedies. The ailments are grouped by bodily systems, but you may find that you need to look in more than one section to find the selection of treatments that will work for you.

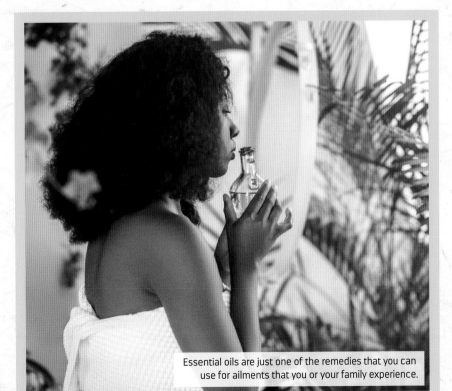

Essential oils are just one of the remedies that you can use for ailments that you or your family experience.

MIND AND EMOTIONS

MENTALLY, WE ARE ALL AFFECTED BY THE SITUATIONS THAT SURROUND US.
Sometimes this can become overwhelming, and we can suffer from stress. If you regularly suffer
from insomnia, depression, anxiety, feeling foggy-headed, dizziness, nausea, feeling drained of
energy, or suffer from persistent bacterial and viral infections, it's time to act. These symptoms of
exhaustion are now widespread and can, at worst, lead to physical collapse.

Diet and physical exercise are both vital for mental health. We really are what we eat. Caffeine,
sugar, and fats can play havoc on our bodies and affect our wellbeing, so think carefully about what
you're eating. If you are having persistent problems, a food sensitivity test might be a good idea,
and an experienced nutritionist may be able to help. You may find that some foods are not being
processed effectively, which can cause you to feel both mentally and physically out of balance. Wheat,

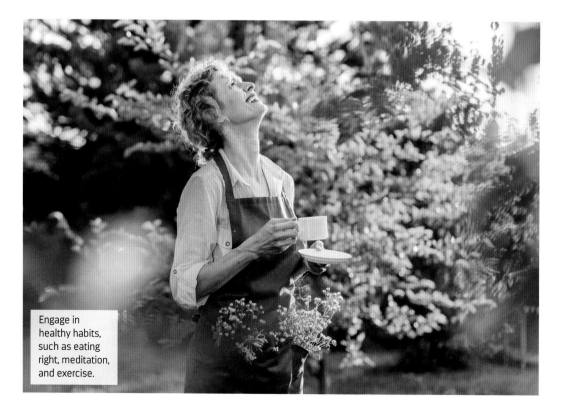

Engage in
healthy habits,
such as eating
right, meditation,
and exercise.

Taking some time to meditate daily will lift your mood, improve your sleep, and generally increase your outlook on life.

yeast, dairy, and sugar are the usual culprits. Try eliminating these from your diet one at a time over the course of a week to check how your body reacts to these foods. Be sure to include plenty of fresh greens, nuts, seeds, and protein to help keep your body healthy while eliminating toxins.

Introducing regular, gentle exercise is another important step towards a happier, healthier mind. Aerobic exercise releases feel-good hormones—known as endorphins—which leave you feeling much brighter after a burst of activity. Be aware that the information we feed ourselves with affects us too—if you can, avoid the newspaper and news programs full of doom and gloom about the state of the world. Choose to read something inspirational or watch an uplifting film instead.

Meditation can be very beneficial in ensuring good mental health and you may find that regular practice helps to improve concentration and memory. Your general mood should lift, sleep will be deeper and more regular, and problems will seem less insurmountable. Bach Flower Remedies have been specially formulated to treat emotional disorders. The blend of five flower essences, Rescue Remedy, is a good place to start as it can be used to treat so many differing conditions. Use it when you are feeling low or anxious.

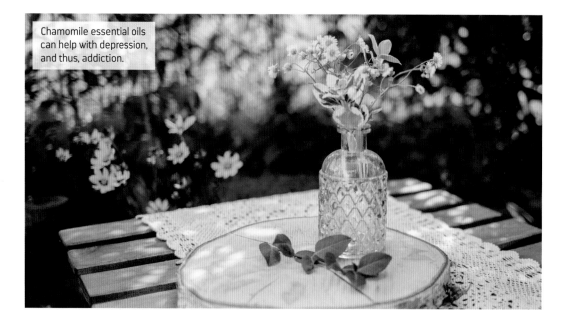

Chamomile essential oils can help with depression, and thus, addiction.

Addiction

Addiction is a dependence on a substance such as alcohol or nicotine. Physical withdrawal symptoms can include cravings, mood swings, and depression. Try using anti-depressant oils such as chamomile, ylang ylang, and clary sage. A few drops of each can be added to a carrier oil such as organic sweet almond oil. Use this to massage into your arms, chest, and legs. It can also be added to a warm bath for an uplifting treat. Also, you might like to add a few drops of clary sage to your cuffs and collar when getting dressed to help you carry the scent with you and allow you to feel the effects all day long. Oats are a useful remedy for helping you to strengthen your willpower when letting something go from your life. They also have a calming effect on the mind. Make oat water (recipe below) and drink three times a day.

Oat Water

Mentally, this is good for strengthening willpower, and physically it can be used to treat the symptoms of diarrhea and cystitis.

- 1 tablespoon oats
- 1 cup water

1. Combine the oats and water in a bowl, stir, and leave to infuse for twenty minutes.

2. Stir again and strain the mixture through a muslin cloth.

3. Drink the resulting liquid. The muslin cloth containing the oats can be tied and used as a bath bag to soothe the skin and to calm the mind and aid more restful sleep.

Anxiety

Anxiety is a state of fear or apprehension that can become constant. It is associated with depression and causes symptoms such as sweaty palms, rapid pulse, breathlessness, headaches, and loss of appetite. Oat can be used as a gentle nerve tonic. Eat porridge for breakfast to benefit from their effects. Also try oat water (page opposite). This tonic can be taken three times a day to help you get over challenging times. Use Rescue Remedy during panic attacks. Place a few drops on the tongue or rub into the pulse points.

Nurturing Tea

Try this calming, nurturing tea when you are feeling low.

- Motherwort, as needed
- Lemon balm, as needed

1. Pick equal amounts of motherwort and lemon balm. Spread on a baking tray and leave in a warm, dry place for one week.

2. Once dried, crumble into a glass jar and store.

3. To drink, place 2 teaspoons of the dried herbs into a cup. Fill with boiling water and leave to infuse for ten minutes. Strain and drink.

Memory Loss

Also known as amnesia, this is a partial or complete memory loss, caused by a physical or mental disease or sometimes from a physical trauma such as a blow to the head. While anyone experiencing memory loss should consult a medical professional, rosemary can help to refresh the memory in minor cases when used in cooking or making an herbal tea.

Rosemary Tea

To refresh the memory in minor cases. Also good for use before exams as it is believed to keep the mind sharp.

- 1 heaped tablespoon chopped fresh (or dried) rosemary
- 1 cup water just off the boil

1. Place rosemary in a cup.

2. Cover with water just off the boil (not boiling) and leave to infuse for ten minutes.

3. Strain and drink. Enjoy up to three cups a day.

Depression

Often triggered by a stressful life event, depression is a feeling of despondency and unhappiness that lasts for a long time. Some women experience this after childbirth when it is known as Post Natal Depression. Borage (also known as starflower) is recognized for its uplifting properties. A tincture can be made from the bright blue flowers.

Borage Tincture

This tincture can help to lift the spirits when everything seems hopeless.

- Handful of borage flowers
- 7 fluid ounces (200 ml) alcohol, such as organic vodka or brandy
- 3½ fluid ounces (100 ml) water

1. Place the borage flowers in a large glass jar with a well-fitting lid.

2. Cover with the alcohol and water.

3. Replace the lid and leave to infuse for two weeks, gently shaking from time to time.

4. Strain the mixture through a muslin cloth, retaining the liquid. Bottle the tincture and store.

5. To drink, add 1 teaspoon to a glass of water.

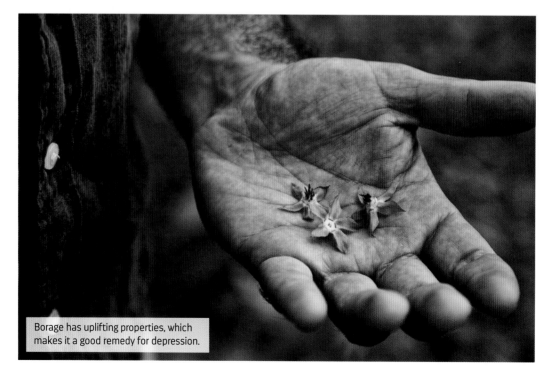

Borage has uplifting properties, which makes it a good remedy for depression.

Yoga Nidra, a yogic sleep, can help you settle down before going to bed.

Insomnia

This refers to the inability to sleep or disturbance of sleep patterns. Can be caused by emotional stress, worry, and exhaustion. Excess caffeine, rich food, and alcohol can also play a part in disturbed sleep patterns. There are plenty of suggestions for helping the mind to rest before sleep but one of the most effective is to keep a notepad by the bed and to jot down whatever is occupying the mind before sleep. I find that this can act as a sort of internal brain cleanse; getting everything out and onto paper so that my mind is ready to let go and go to sleep.

A short yoga practice using calming poses such as shoulder stand followed by a relaxation called Yoga Nidra can also help to promote restful sleep. Yoga Nidra is known as the yogic sleep and is deeply relaxing to the mind and body. It is a great way to settle before drifting off at night. You can also use the power of mustard and take a hot footbath before bed to help calm the mind (see recipe on page 75). The mustard draws blood away from the head, aiding relaxation.

Herbal Bath Bag

Make this herbal bath bag for a soak just before bed, which should help you get a good night's rest.

- 1 tablespoon dried chamomile flowers
- 1 tablespoon dried lavender flowers
- 1 tablespoon oats

1. Take an 11½-inch (30 cm) square of muslin and lay it out flat.

2. Place the dried flowers and oats in the center of the muslin square. Gather up the corners and tie with string to secure.

3. Place in a warm bath and relax.

Obsessive-Compulsive Disorder (OCD)

The essential oils chamomile and marjoram can be burned to help you find balance.

Obsessive-compulsive disorder is an obsession to perform a certain ritual. This can be something as simple as repeated hand washing or repeated checking that the windows are shut at night, for example. It usually starts after a stressful life event, and minor obsessions and compulsions are said to affect fifteen percent of the population.

Chamomile is a good herb to help calm the mind, release tension, and encourage a release of behavioral patterns. Use as a tea and drink as often as needed throughout the day. Burn the essential oil of chamomile in an oil burner along with marjoram, both of which are helpful in encouraging you to find balance. You can also add a few drops of each to a warm relaxing bath.

Chamomile Tea

Chamomile has a relaxing effect, which can be helpful for managing stress and improving sleep.

- 1 heaped tablespoon chamomile flowers (or chamomile teabag)
- 1 cup water just off the boil

1. Place chamomile in a cup.
2. Cover with water just off the boil (not boiling) and leave to infuse for ten minutes.
3. Strain and drink. Enjoy up to three cups a day.

Relaxing Bath Blend

This soothing bath blend can be used to ease mental distress.

- 3 drops Roman chamomile essential oil
- 6 drops sweet marjoram essential oil
- ½ cup carrier oil, such as sweet almond, or even olive oil

1. Mix the oils in a bowl or glass jar.
2. Run a warm bath.
3. Add your oil blend to running water. Step in and soak for at least fifteen minutes.

Phobias

This is a fear of something that can cause disruption to everyday living. Agoraphobia (fear of open spaces) and acrophobia (fear of heights) are some of the more common phobias, but they can range from fear of another person or an object to any number of experiences or situations. It is said that ten percent of the population have a phobia of one kind or another.

The flower essences created by Dr. Bach were developed to help people deal with emotional problems and there are several remedies that can help with phobias. Rescue Remedy, for example, can be used to treat causes of mild to severe panic—place five drops on the tongue, or apply to pulse points on the wrist and behind the ears.

Aromatherapy can be very beneficial in the treatment of phobias. A blend of essential oils such as bergamot, lavender, melissa, and ylang ylang can be calming and rebalancing to the nervous system when in a state of distress. Add a few drops of each to a carrier oil to make up a bath blend. It will have a slight sedative effect.

Fear Diffuser

This can be spritzed as often as necessary during challenging times.

- A few drops of bergamot, lavender, melissa, and ylang ylang essential oils
- Spring water, as needed

1. Take a small spray-top bottle and add a few drops of each essential oil.
2. Top up with spring water.
3. Spritz over the face (close your eyes) and wrists as needed.

Fear-Busting Bath Blend

When you are feeling particularly nervous or distressed, add this bath blend to a warm tub and soak for at least twenty minutes.

- 6 drops lavender essential oil
- 5 drops bergamot essential oil
- 4 drops lemon balm essential oil
- 3 drops ylang ylang essential oil
- ½ cup carrier oil, such as sweet almond or even olive oil

1. Mix the oils in a bowl or glass jar.
2. Run a warm bath.
3. Add your oil blend to running water.
4. Step in and soak for at least twenty minutes.

Stress

Stress is a growing disorder in our modern world. Many factors can affect our mental health, such as inadequate diet, environment, noise pollution, and financial strains. This mental discomfort has a knock-on effect on the body, encouraging a rapid production of hormones, which can cause increased breathing and heart rate, leading to nausea and tense muscles.

As soon as the stressful situation is resolved, the body returns to normal. If the situation continues, energy levels dwindle and exhaustion sets in. Fortunately, there are many natural treatments for this common disorder. The first and most obvious is to take a good look at your life and address the common triggers for stress. Are you putting in longer and longer hours at work? Do you feel that your responsibilities at home are too great with children to care for, a house to keep tidy, and a household to run? Make a list of things that stress you out—school run, cooking for the family, monthly reports at work, for example.

Acknowledging these stressful situations is the first step in dealing with them. Once you have a list of stressful things in your life, take the first item on your list and brainstorm who or what could support you. Perhaps your neighbor could take the children to school, and you could collect them. Maybe you could have a picnic supper at the weekends, or a takeaway night, or perhaps someone else in your household could take over the cooking for a while. The monthly reports might be a task that could be completed by a colleague. Stick this list up in a prominent place and start to action the

Sip hot herbal tea to help reduce stress.

alternatives. There are also several natural remedies that can support you in this process. Starting the day with a bowl of porridge helps to strengthen the system and gives you a clearer and more positive outlook. Or, bathe with a few drops of essential oils to wash your troubles away.

Stress-Away Bath Blend

For those days when you need a little extra support, try this soothing and uplifting bath blend. Don't worry if you don't have all the essential oils on hand. Work with what you do have (e.g., a blend of rose, lavender, and neroli smells divine and works wonders).

- 7 drops rose otto essential oil
- 6 drops geranium essential oil
- 5 drops lavender essential oil
- 4 drops Roman chamomile essential oil
- 3 drops neroli essential oil
- ½ cup carrier oil, such as sweet almond or even olive oil
- 1 cup Epsom salts

1. Mix the oils and salt in a large bowl or large Kilner jar.

2. Run a warm bath.

3. Add your blend to running water.

4. Step in and soak for at least twenty minutes.

Ten Tips to De-Stress

Here are some ideas for when the going gets tough. Always try to remember that tomorrow is another day. If all else fails, get an early night and wake up with a fresh take on life.

1. Wake up early in the morning to enjoy half an hour of quiet time on your own. This will allow you time to collect your thoughts and energize yourself for the day ahead.

2. Go for a bracing walk. Exercise releases serotonin, the happy hormone, so you start to feel better as soon as you get into your stride.

3. Arrange a night in with your partner. Using some sensual essential oils, give each other a massage.

4. Breathe properly. Many of us use only one-tenth of our lung capacity. Imagine how good we would feel if we learned to use half or more? Breath work can teach us how to use more of our lungs' full potential.

5. Run a warm bath, surround it with candles, climb in, and relax.

6. Laugh. Phone a friend who makes you laugh, or rent a funny movie.

7. Retreat to a quiet place, such as a favorite armchair, and enjoy a good book.

8. Take your family out for the day. Getting away from the house and the daily routine of chores does everyone a world of good occasionally.

9. Take an evening course in something you feel passionate about.

10. If all hell is breaking loose and you feel your stress levels rising, walk into another room and count slowly to ten before returning to salvage the situation.

We all know of the classic rose flower, but a rose has many healing properties other than smelling good.

Plant Profile: Rose

The rose is an uplifting and sensual plant. Lovers have recognized this beautiful, perfumed flower since ancient times—Cleopatra was said to have strewn the floor with rose petals when she invited Mark Anthony into her boudoir. Today, couples can use roses to encourage love and communication. Try bathing together in a bathtub filled with rose petals and a few drops of rose essential oil. Or make your own massage blend. Rose petals make an alluring addition to a warm bath and a handful thrown under running water can actually help to alleviate rheumatic pains. Sore, tired eyes can be soothed using an infusion, made by steeping a few rose petals in hot water.

Lovers' Massage Oil

Create a special oil that you can use to massage each other with to soothe and reconnect.

- 3.3 ounces (100 ml) sweet almond oil
- 4 drops rose otto essential oil
- 4 drops ylang ylang essential oil

1. Place the sweet almond oil in a dark bottle.

2. Add the essential oils to the carrier oil and use as needed to massage long, sweeping strokes across each other's bodies, focusing on tight areas such as the shoulders and upper back. Avoid pressing directly on the spine.

3. Always check that the pressure is okay for your massage recipient.

Soothing Eye Bath

Make an infusion with rose petals to soothe tired eyes.

- 6–7 rose petals
- 1 cup hot water

1. Add rose petals to a cup of hot water.

2. Allow to steep and cool to tepid. Strain to remove petals.

3. Soak a clean muslin cloth or cotton eye pad in the warm water. Apply directly to the eye. Can be made fresh and applied several times a day.

Many natural toiletries use the power and scent of rose, and rose oil is often used as a perfume. It is one of the world's most expensive commodities, weight by weight worth more than gold. Aromatherapists value it for its uplifting and soothing properties, especially for nervous tension. When the blooms fade and the petals fall away, the plant bears a fruit called a hip, containing seeds, which are rich in Vitamin C. They also contain B vitamins and a high amount of carotene. During WWII, due to a shortage of fruit and vegetables, children were encouraged to pick rose hips on their way to school so that they could be boiled up to make a nutritive syrup, which was issued as a dietary supplement.

Rosehips are excellent for the skin, can help to prevent infection, and are also a known blood purifier. The Chinese use rosehip tea to relieve stomachache and to regulate vital energy. This tea can also be blended with a pinch of cloves and cinnamon to stimulate and restore the system. It is best to avoid drinking this tea late at night, as rosehips stimulate the adrenal glands.

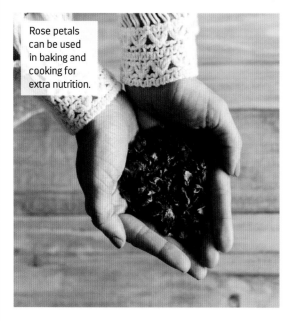

Rose petals can be used in baking and cooking for extra nutrition.

In cooking, rose petals have been used for centuries to add elegance as well as for added nutrition. Try tossing a few petals into a fruit salad, or as a cake decoration. Rosehips can be used to make a fine hedgerow wine, jams, jellies, syrups, tarts, breads, and in many other forms of baking. They impart a good color and a subtle sweetness to many dishes. To harness the healing powers of the rosehip as the Chinese do, without the use of a great deal of sugar that is needed to produce a syrup, try making rosehip tea (see page 51).

Nervous System

A LITTLE STRESS CAN BE HEALTHY FOR THE HEART AND MIND. HOWEVER, IT IS easy for us to tip over the edge into anxiety, panic, and even depression. Stress affects the whole person, physically, mentally, and emotionally. This is why holistic therapies are such a powerful weapon against the effects of stress as they work on all levels to try and bring you back into balance, body, mind, and spirit.

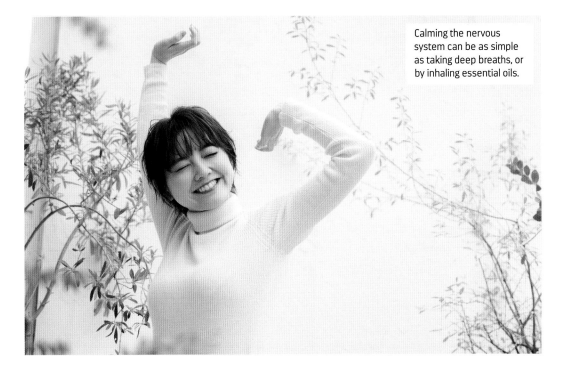

Calming the nervous system can be as simple as taking deep breaths, or by inhaling essential oils.

Multiple Sclerosis

Multiple sclerosis is a chronic disease of the nervous system that affects the sheaths of the nerves, which become inflamed, leading to gradual loss of nerve function. The disease is characterized by its cycle of remission and relapse. Practicing yoga can help prevent further deterioration of the disorder as it improves flexibility of the limbs and prevents stiffness.

Practicing yoga can prevent deterioration caused by multiple sclerosis.

Regular massage of the joints is helpful, as is water therapy. At home, try hot mineral baths with Epsom salts, alternating between hot and cold showers to help stimulate the nerves twice a day. Add raw dairy and cultured products to the diet such as raw unsalted butter (preferably organic and from grass-fed cows), homemade cottage cheese, and unfiltered honey. Increase intake of gamma-linoleic acid found in safflower and evening primrose oil. Rescue Remedy can be used to help ease the symptoms and relieve anxiety.

Epsom Salts Bath

A bath with Epsom salts (magnesium sulphate) is thought to ease pain and relieve inflammation, making it beneficial to treat sore muscles, reduce swelling, and ease migraine symptoms.

- 1 cup Epsom salts

1. Add the salts to a warm (not too hot) bath.

2. Relax and enjoy for at least twenty minutes.

3. If you are comfortable and able to, you can finish off with a cool (not too cold) shower to activate the circulatory system.

Stroke

A stroke is a condition where a blood clot or ruptured artery or blood vessel interrupts blood flow to an area of the brain. A lack of oxygen and glucose flowing to the brain causes damage, often resulting in impaired speech, movement, and memory. Smaller strokes may result in minor problems, such as weakness in an arm or leg. Larger strokes may lead to paralysis.

Many stroke patients are left with weakness on one side of the body, difficulty speaking, incontinence, and bladder problems. Gently massage the body daily especially the paralyzed muscles. Use a carrier oil such as organic sweet almond oil with a few drops of rosemary essential oil.

Yarrow or Rosemary Tea

Both yarrow and rosemary can both to improve circulation.

- 1 handful yarrow leaves or 3 small sprigs rosemary
- Boiling water, as needed

1. Place the yarrow or rosemary in a cup and add boiling water.
2. Place a plate over the top and leave to infuse for ten minutes.
3. Strain and drink up to three cups daily.

Parkinson's Disease

Parkinson's disease is a serious chronic disease of the nervous system causing continuous tremors or shaking and stiffness of the neck. Oats are calming and strengthening to the nervous system. You can make your own nerve tonic to drink regularly throughout the day.

Nerve Tonic

- 1 tablespoon oats
- ½ pint (300 ml) water

1. Place the oats and water in a saucepan.
2. Bring to a boil and simmer for five minutes.
3. Strain and drink as needed.

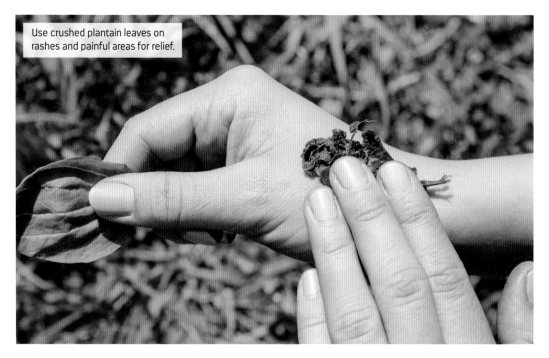

Use crushed plantain leaves on rashes and painful areas for relief.

Shingles

Shingles is a painful disease caused by the herpes zoster virus (chicken pox). Symptoms can include sensitivity in the affected area, high fever, sickness, and a painful rash of small blisters. Use crushed plantain leaves to soothe neuralgic pains and rash. Crush the leaves and apply to the affected area. Reapply as often as needed. Bathe the infected area with diluted tincture of calendula (see page 116), plantain or St. John's Wort. Dilute one part to ten parts water, soak a cloth, and apply a cold compress to the affected area.

Plantain Tincture

- 1 large handful plantain leaves
- 7 fluid ounces (200 ml) alcohol, such as organic vodka
- 3½ fluid ounces (100 ml) water

1. Place the plantain leaves in a large glass jar and cover with the alcohol and water.

2. Put on the lid and leave for two weeks, shaking occasionally.

3. Strain the liquid through a sieve with a muslin cloth over it.

4. Pour the liquid into a dark glass bottle and store for up to a year.

Migraine

A migraine is a severe headache that generally occurs on one side of the head. It is associated with disorders of digestion, liver, and vision. Migraines usually occur when a person is under great mental tension. The pain lasts around three days, and may be accompanied by nausea and vomiting. Eye disturbances can occur such as intolerance of light, blurred vision, black spots or zigzag lines that appear before the eyes, or partly blank vision. The headache is usually accompanied by weakness in an arm or leg and tingly and numb feeling.

Patients tend to be compulsive workers with overworked and continuously stressed head and neck muscles. Apply a cold compress to the head and face. Feverfew is a plant that can be used to treat migraine. Eat two small leaves with food.

Compress for Migraine Attacks

Use when you feel an attack coming on to calm the system and alleviate the pain.

- 2 drops lavender essential oil
- Cool water, as needed

1. Fill a bowl with cool water.
2. Add the lavender essential oil.
3. Soak a cotton cloth in the water, wring out, and apply to the temples.

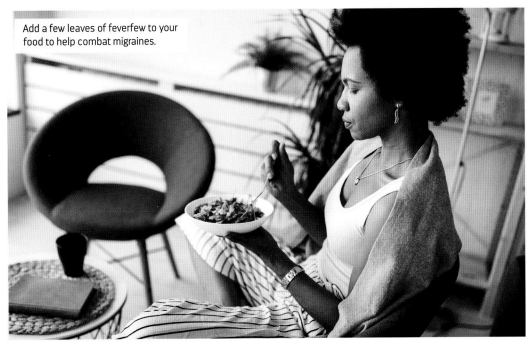

Add a few leaves of feverfew to your food to help combat migraines.

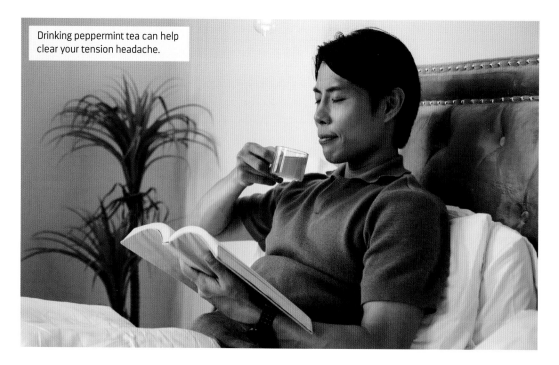

Drinking peppermint tea can help clear your tension headache.

Headache

A headache indicates that something is wrong somewhere in the body. Pain arises from irritation to the nerve endings in the shoulder, neck, and scalp muscles and in smooth muscles encircling the blood vessels. A ginger root footbath can help to ease the pain and warm the body. A mustard footbath can also be helpful (see page 75). Drink peppermint tea to calm and soothe the system and help to clear a tension headache. Massage a drop or two of lavender oil into your temples or the pulse points on the wrist. Alternatively, apply a few drops to a handkerchief and inhale regularly to reduce pain. Take a soothing warm bath; swirl in a few drops each of chamomile, lavender, and ylang ylang essential oils.

Comforting Ginger Root Footbath

Ease the pain and warm the body with this nurturing footbath.

- 1 (2-inch) ginger root, grated
- 1 large bowl (big enough to fit both your feet in) of warm water

1. Fill the bowl with water that is warm to the touch.

2. Add grated ginger.

3. Place your feet into the bowl and cover with a towel to keep the water warm. Relax for fifteen minutes.

Neuralgia

Neuralgia describes any pain that originates in the nerve. The pain may be intermittent or continuous. St. John's Wort is a traditional herbal remedy for nerve damage. Use the oil to gently massage the body.

St. John's Wort Oil

This oil can be used for massage to help heal nerve damage. It is also useful for treating skin complaints such as cold sores.

- 1 handful flowering tops from the St. John's Wort plant
- 7 fluid ounces (200 ml) sunflower oil

1. Place the flowering tops in a pestle with a little of the oil.

2. Pound together until you have a mash and put the mashed flowers into a large glass jar. Cover with more oil.

3. Shake well and leave in direct sunlight for twenty-one days. The oil will turn red when it is ready for use.

Epilepsy

Epilepsy is a serious disease of the central nervous system which presents as repeated fits or attacks of unconsciousness with often violent shivers. Attacks generally reduce with age, but the uncertainty in the time of attack is one major problem. Avoid physical and mental stress. Take a warm Epsom salts bath once a day and take Rescue Remedy as you feel an attack coming on.

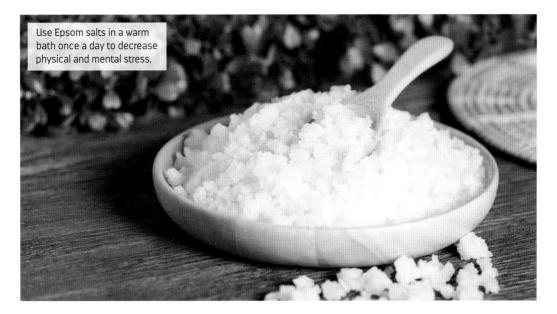

Use Epsom salts in a warm bath once a day to decrease physical and mental stress.

Plant Profile: Rosemary

Rosemary is a multipurpose herb—its leaves, flowers, and essential oil can be used in a variety of ways including culinary, medicinal, and in aromatherapy. It is a hardy, shrubby perennial bush that grows up to 1½ yards (1.5 meters) high with green-grey needle-shaped evergreen leaves and pale blue-lilac flowers that attract bees. It originates from Asia, but is now cultivated widely in many herb gardens in the West.

Growing rosemary is relatively easy. Depending on your climate, rosemary can be planted in the garden as a border plant or single ornamental. It likes sun and good drainage, and does very well in hot or dry climates. It will tolerate freezing temperatures for a short time if it's protected from cold winds. During long, cold winters, cultivate in a pot that can be brought inside and left in a sunny window or greenhouse. Rosemary grows well in most soils, but thrives as a more fragrant plant in a more alkaline soil; so add ground eggshells or wood ash if your soil tends to the acidic side.

The name is derived from the Latin *rosmarinus* or "sea dew", as it loves water. The Egyptians, Hebrews, Greeks, and Romans considered the herb to be sacred, and even in the Middle Ages it was used to ward off evil spirits and used as a protection against the plague. Rosemary was an essential part of the apothecary's repertoire during the Renaissance and the French regarded it as a miraculous cure-all.

Because rosemary was easily harvested from the wild, it was used as an incense by the poor as a substitute for expensive frankincense- or myrrh-based incense in ancient Greece and Rome. When a twig of rosemary is burned, it is said to rid space of negativity because of its cleansing vibrations. It was burnt at shrines in Ancient Greece to drive away evil spirits and illnesses.

Hippocrates, Galen, and Dioscorides all prescribed rosemary for liver problems. Rosemary is an astringent, restorative herb that is excellent for muscle

Rosemary essential oil has a stimulating effect on the brain and central nervous systems.

aches and strains and rheumatism. It increases the rate of perspiration while stimulating the liver and gallbladder. It improves digestion and circulation and has antibacterial, antifungal, antiviral, analgesic, antidepressant, and anti-inflammatory properties. It is an outstanding free radical scavenger and therefore has amazing antioxidant

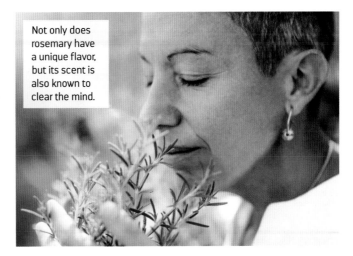

Not only does rosemary have a unique flavor, but its scent is also known to clear the mind.

properties. It has a tightening, stimulating effect on the skin and is a wonderful treatment for the hair and scalp.

Rosemary essential oil is extracted from the fresh flowering tops by steam distillation and has a clear, powerful, and refreshing herbal smell. It can be used in vaporizers and oil burners, in the bath or in a carrier oil for massage directly onto the skin. It has a highly stimulating action and because of this it may not be suitable for people with epilepsy or high blood pressure and should also not be used during pregnancy. It has a pronounced stimulating effect on the brain and central nervous system and is great for clearing the mind, improving memory, and mental awareness.

The diuretic properties of rosemary oil are useful for reducing water retention caused by premenstrual tension and menstruation, and for obesity and cellulite. It is also effective for asthma, bronchitis, catarrh, sinus problems, and whooping cough. On the skin, it helps to ease congestion, puffiness, and swelling and can also be used for acne, dermatitis, and eczema.

Rosemary is a great thirst quencher and adding rosemary to your tea creates a unique flavor that is good for a pick-me-up. Pick a 4-inch (10-cm) sprig, wash it, add to your teapot, and steep for two to three minutes. The tea can be served with or without milk.

Adding rosemary to marinades adds a refreshing, uplifting flavor. Add two teaspoons of crushed rosemary leaves to every two tablespoons of olive oil. Throw in a dash of tamari sauce and brush over butternut squash, mushrooms, or potatoes and leave to marinade before baking or barbecuing. The flowers can also be added to salads.

DIGESTIVE SYSTEM

DID YOU KNOW THAT SEVENTY PERCENT OF YOUR IMMUNE SYSTEM LIVES IN THE gut? Were you aware that stomach acid, far from being a negative element, is a protective barrier, killing harmful bacteria? And did you realize that it's not just food, but lifestyle as well that helps you maintain a healthy acid/alkaline balance so that you can process your food efficiently for maximum wellbeing? Taking care of your digestive system means ensuring that you eat regular meals, rather than skipping meals or just having a coffee in the morning for breakfast.

Try eating smaller meals more regularly, eating earlier in the evening, and not drinking too much water with meals, as this can dilute the gastric juices. Avoid rich, fatty food that is challenging for your digestive system to cope with, and take care with things like fizzy drinks, which can be very acidic and irritating to the stomach lining. Relaxation should be an important part of your eating routine. Don't eat while stressed. The digestion can be "turned off" by the fight-or-flight stress response. It is better to wait until you are calm so that the body is in a better state to receive food. Eating at a table with friends and family is a far healthier way for the body to receive nutrients than slumped in front of the TV.

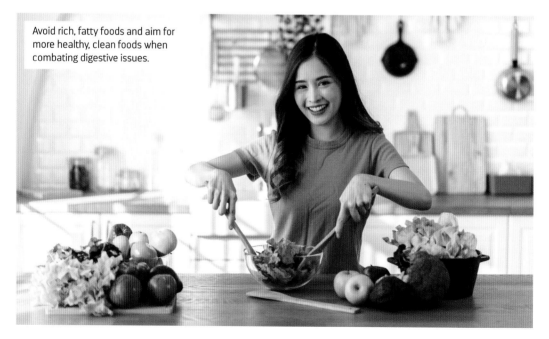

Avoid rich, fatty foods and aim for more healthy, clean foods when combating digestive issues.

Stomach acid is a necessary part of digestion, though it is often seen as a bad thing, to be controlled by antacids or acid-blocking drugs. In fact, many nutritionists see clients that have the opposite problem—they have too little stomach acid, which can also cause problems with indigestion. Herbs are excellent at healing stomach complaints. They can help balance excess acid, soothe inflamed mucus membranes, and protect against the damage caused by many orthodox medications.

Stomach ulcers are becoming very common in younger, seemingly fit and healthy individuals. Stress, caffeine, overeating, erratic eating patterns, bad diet, and not drinking

Dried herbs heal stomach issues in many ways, like balancing excess acid.

enough water all lead to heat in the stomach causing ulceration. Traditional Chinese medicine calls this "Stomach fire" as it literally feels like the stomach is on fire, with burning sensations, bleeding gums, constant hunger, bad breath, and sluggish bowels. If these symptoms appear, even in a mild form, action must be taken. Spicy and fried foods, red meat, alcohol, citrus fruit, tomatoes, caffeine, and tobacco will aggravate and make it very difficult for the stomach lining to heal. There are many alternative ways of dealing with stomach-related imbalances.

The liver is another important organ in the digestive system; it governs the digestive process and is responsible for regulating, cleaning, and storing the blood in the body. It is our largest organ and is filled with blood. The better condition our liver is in, the better it can ensure that the blood that circulates around our bodies nourishes our muscles and keeps them supple and pain free. The liver makes bile to emulsify fats for digestion, makes and breaks down hormones, including cholesterol and estrogens, and regulates blood sugar levels. One of its most important roles is detoxification. The liver manufactures 13,000 chemicals and has 2,000 enzyme systems critical to the smooth operation of our bodies and minds. Nearly all vitamins and minerals that we need are enzymatically processed by the liver before we can use them.

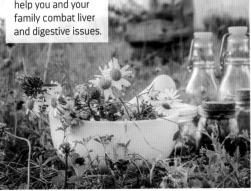
Cultivating medicinal herbs in your garden can help you and your family combat liver and digestive issues.

Some of the symptoms of liver problems are poor digestion, abdominal bloating, nausea after fatty foods, unstable blood sugar levels, waking with bad breath and/or coated tongue, intolerance to greasy/fatty foods, constipation, fatigue and sleepiness after eating, yellow whites of eyes, yellowish color of skin, lowered tolerance to alcohol, and excessive body heat. If you suspect an imbalance in your liver, look out for a dip in energy in the late afternoon which leads to a craving for chocolate or something sweet, waking in the early hours of the morning and being unable to drop back off to sleep because of an overactive mind, unusual irritability over issues which do not generally cause such a reaction, or skin and digestive problems.

Fortunately, there are several natural remedies that can be used to treat disorders of the digestive system. Find out how to improve your digestion using herbs such as fennel and dill, treat stomachache with rosehip tea, and get things moving again in cases of constipation.

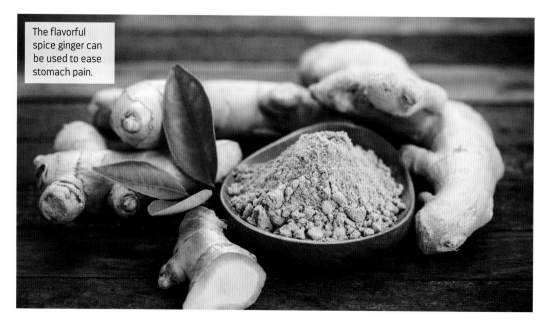

The flavorful spice ginger can be used to ease stomach pain.

Nausea and Vomiting

Nausea and vomiting is a symptom of many disorders including migraine, food poisoning, and gastroenteritis. Stress and anxiety can cause feelings of nausea without vomiting. Ginger tea can be drunk to warm and ease stomach pain, especially when traveling causes nausea. It is also useful in cases of morning sickness during pregnancy. Rescue remedy can be used, and it will help calm the mind and soothe the body. Take five drops in a glass of water as needed.

Warming Ginger Tea

- ½ thumb sixed knob of ginger, grated (or ¼ teaspoon dried ginger)
- Boiling water, as needed

1. Grate the ginger into a cup.

2. Cover with boiling water and leave to infuse for ten minutes.

3. Strain and drink. Enjoy up to three cups a day.

Gastroenteritis

Gastroenteritis is acute inflammation of the stomach caused by bacteria or a virus. Fever usually accompanies with diarrhea and abdominal pain. A teaspoon of honey taken every few hours will act as a natural antibiotic and is anti-inflammatory. It will also keep the body's strength up at a challenging time. Massage essential oil of Roman chamomile into the abdomen area to ease discomfort. Take a tablespoon of live yogurt three times a day when the symptoms start to ease, to repopulate the gut with healthy flora.

Stomachache

The Chinese make a tea from rosehips to alleviate stomachaches. This tea also helps to regulate vital energy as it stimulates the adrenal glands—avoid late at night for this reason. To harness the healing powers of the rosehip without the use of a great deal of sugar needed to produce a syrup, try making rosehip tea.

Vital Energy-Boosting Rosehip Tea

Make a tea from rosehips that has traditionally been used to boost energy and relieve stomachaches.

- 4 teaspoons rosehips, crushed
- 4 cups water

1. Place the rosehips and water in a pan over a medium heat. Boil for twenty minutes.
2. Strain thoroughly (using a muslin cloth) to remove any irritating hairs.
3. Keep warm in a thermos and enjoy throughout the day. Avoid drinking too close to bedtime because of the effect on the adrenal system.

Travel Sickness

Sensitivity to motion when traveling can cause feelings of nausea and sickness. Take a flask of chamomile, peppermint, or fennel tea with you to sip throughout the journey. Chew fresh peppermint leaves to settle the stomach. (Also see Peppermint Infusion on page 55.)

Indigestion and Heartburn

Indigestion and heartburn can cause discomfort in the abdomen, often after eating rich food or eating too quickly. Drink peppermint tea to soothe the stomach and aid digestion. You can also rub essential oil of peppermint into the stomach to ease discomfort. Fennel seeds eaten after a meal can help the stomach to digest rich foods. Make an infusion of dill to reduce pains from trapped gas. Drink fresh cucumber juice or eat a cucumber to reduce the effects of heartburn or acid reflex.

Dill Infusion

- 1 handful dill
- Boiling water, as needed

1. Place dill in a cup. Cover with boiling water and place a plate over the top.
2. Leave to infuse for ten minutes.
3. Strain and drink while still warm.

Constipation

Constipation is painful or irregular bowel movements caused by compacted matter in the colon. Massage rosemary or fennel oil into the abdomen in a clockwise direction to follow the movement of the colon. Certain herbs have a laxative effect and should be used with care but can help relieve the body. Licorice is one such herb, which can be made into an infusion and drunk as needed, up to three cups per day.

Licorice Infusion

- 1 stick licorice
- Boiling water, as needed

1. Place licorice, broken into pieces, into a cup. Cover with boiling water and place a plate on top.
2. Leave to infuse for ten minutes.
3. Strain through a tea strainer and drink as required.

Diarrhea

Diarrhea, or loose runny stools, are the result of many illnesses. It can also be caused by stress or anxiety. Oats are a soothing, binding food that can aid gut health. Make some oat water (see page 28), and drink three times a day. Carrot juice is a traditional remedy for diarrhea, especially for babies. You can also make a carrot soup to soothe the bowels.

Carrot Juice

- 3 carrots

1. Juice carrots in a juicer.
2. Pour into a glass and drink immediately.
3. Drink three times a day while symptoms persist.

Irritable Bowel Syndrome (IBS)

Irritable bowel syndrome is a common disorder with abdominal pain and diarrhea alternating with constipation. Drink soothing herbal teas of peppermint and chamomile, which all have anti-spasmodic properties. Massage Roman chamomile essential oil into the abdomen.

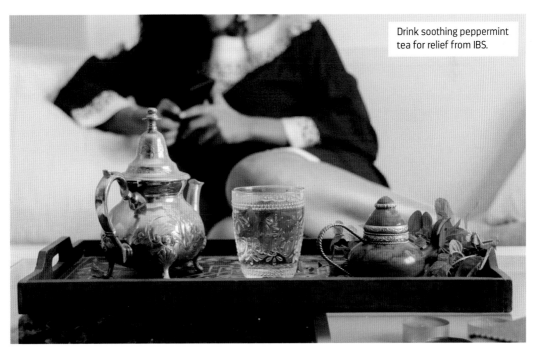

Drink soothing peppermint tea for relief from IBS.

Flatulence

This is an excessive amount of gas in the body, often caused by eating foods that disagree with the digestive system or eating too quickly. Eat celery seeds to reduce flatulence. Make a dill infusion (see page 52) to ease any discomfort.

Hepatitis

Hepatitis means inflammation (*itis*) of the liver (*hepar*)—an irritation or swelling of the liver cells. There are many causes of hepatitis, including viral infections. Most of us will have heard of types A, B, and C, but the variations also include autoimmune hepatitis, fatty liver hepatitis, alcoholic hepatitis, and toxin-induced hepatitis. It is estimated that around 250 million people globally are affected by hepatitis C. Moreover, an estimated 400 million people are chronic carriers of hepatitis B. Liver tonics, such as milk thistle, dandelion, and nettle can be taken daily to help healing. Massage chamomile or grapefruit essential oils into the abdomen or take a warm bath with a few drops of either added.

Love Your Liver Tincture

Take this tincture daily to promote healing.

- 1 ounce dried milk thistle seeds
- 1 ounce dried nettle leaves
- ½ ounce dried dandelion root
- 12½ ounces 100-proof alcohol

1. Coarsely grind milk thistle seeds in a coffee grinder.

2. Add thistle, dandelion, and nettle to a large jar. Pour alcohol in so it covers all the herbs.

3. Seal and shake well. Store in a dark place at room temperature. Allow to steep for at least three weeks.

4. When you're ready, strain and pour tincture into dark bottles. Can take ½ teaspoon a day.

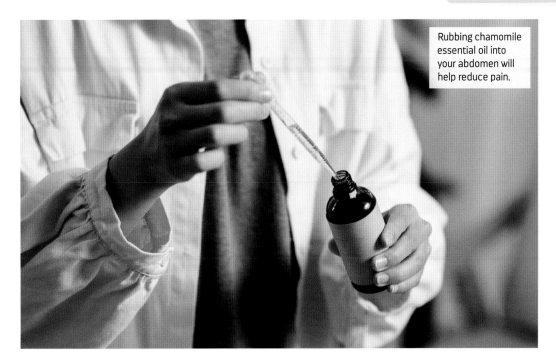

Rubbing chamomile essential oil into your abdomen will help reduce pain.

Crohn's Disease

Crohn's disease is inflammation of the bowel, which can cause lower abdominal pain, anemia, and appetite and weight loss. Add a few drops of lavender oil to a warm bath to help you relax. Rub a few drops of chamomile essential oil into the abdomen to soothe pain. Drink an infusion of peppermint to soothe and protect the gut lining from irritation.

Peppermint Infusion

This infusion can also help to ease the symptoms of travel sickness. Make the infusion in a flask and drink as required on your journey.

- 1 handful peppermint leaves
- Boiling water, as needed

1. Place peppermint leaves in a cup. Cover with boiling water and place a plate on top.
2. Leave to infuse for ten minutes.
3. Strain through a tea strainer and drink as required.

Plant Profile: Dandelion

The dandelion (*taraxacum officinale*) is thought to have gotten its name due to the shape of its leaves, the wide teeth likened to lion's teeth (hence *dent-de-lion* in Old French). The plant is considered a weed by many but actually has high nutritive benefits and health-boosting properties. The bane of many gardeners around the world, as fast as you pull the dandelion up, they sprout back, and their taproot grows deep and strong.

This European plant was originally introduced to other continents to provide food for honeybees. Eighty-five different species of insects feast on its pollen, and the seeds are enjoyed by songbirds. The plant is easily recognized, both in the spring and summer with its vibrant yellow ray flowers and in late summer when the seed head appears. The seed head can develop overnight and is composed of hundreds of tiny, parachuted seeds, ready to spread far and wide into the wind to pollinate the plant.

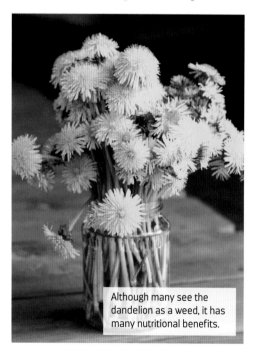

Although many see the dandelion as a weed, it has many nutritional benefits.

When broken, the stem and the root exude a milky, sticky sap that can supposedly remove warts, pimples, and sores. It can also be applied to bee stings and blisters to soothe and calm the inflammation. Despite the concept that dandelion is a bitter plant, the young leaves can be enjoyed raw in salads and other dishes. Today our palate is conditioned to prefer sweet or overly salty foods and to dislike bitter flavors, but in earlier times dandelions were enjoyed regularly. Once you acquire a taste for them, they can enhance a salad, adding a depth to its flavor. Harvest in early spring before the flowers grow. They can also be harvested again in late autumn. Avoid any plants that might have been contaminated by herbicides or pesticides. Sautéed or steamed, dandelions have a much gentler flavor and can be added to soups, stews, and breads.

Liver Tonic Dandelion Decoction

As well as strengthening the whole system, this can also be used to treat hangovers. Don't use too much, as it can have a laxative effect.

- 2 teaspoons dried dandelion root
- 2 cups water

1. Place dandelion root and water in a saucepan and bring to a boil.
2. Allow to simmer for fifteen minutes.
3. Strain into cups and drink a cup as a morning boost.

Dandelion leaves are one of the most nutritious greens available to us. They have a greater concentration of beta-carotene than carrots, are very rich in iron and calcium, and packed with vitamins and minerals. The flowers have traditionally been used to make wine. If you would like to try this, harvest the flowers in mid spring, remove all green parts, and find a recipe on the internet or in a wild food cookbook. The flowers can also brighten up a spring salad, or you can coat them in batter and fry lightly to make golden fritters.

The taproot can be eaten all year round and, although not as tasty as some other wild root vegetables, can be a useful ingredient to bulk out a potato and leek (or other spring vegetable) soup. A beer that acts as a blood purifier and tonic is made in northern England by combining dandelion roots with burdock. A decoction of the taproot is believed to strengthen the body's whole system, especially the liver and gallbladder. Hence it is often used as part of an herbal spring clean for the body. A daily cup of tea made by steeping the leaves in boiling water can help people who are rundown, as it is so rich in vitamins and minerals. It is an excellent digestive aid. This strong tea can also be added to bathwater to soothe inflamed skin and eczema.

Energy-Boosting Dandelion Tea

Take this daily in the springtime if you're feeling rundown. You can also add it to bathwater to treat skin conditions such as eczema.

- 1 tablespoon dandelion flowers (dried or fresh)
- 5 fluid ounces hot water, just off the boil

1. Place dandelion flowers in a cup and add hot water.
2. Cover and allow to steep for ten minutes.
3. Strain and drink. Can be enjoyed throughout the day.

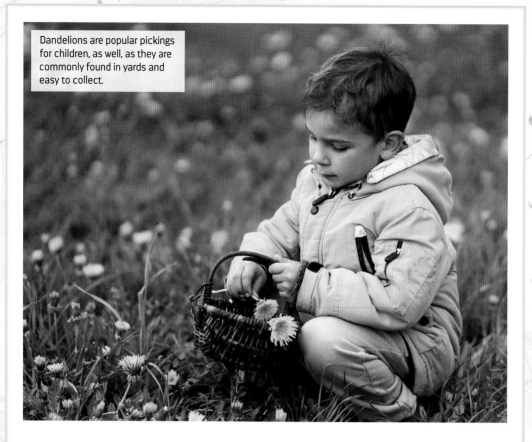

Dandelions are popular pickings for children, as well, as they are commonly found in yards and easy to collect.

During WWI, when natural rubber supplies were cut off, Henry Ford experimented with latex made from dandelions as an alternative. He succeeded in making a high-quality product but had problems in sourcing the quantities that he needed, and the research was abandoned at the end of the war. In Druid lore, to dream of a dandelion is a symbol of difficult times ahead, a period of change and challenge that can have beneficial effect on the dreamer. Children use the seed heads as clocks, and lovers once used the dandelion clock as a divination tool to find out where their partner's devotion lay.

Plant Profile: Milk Thistle

The prickly yet beautiful milk thistle (*Silybum marianum*) is a flowering plant from the Asteraceae, or daisy family. It grows prolifically in Mediterranean countries, North Africa, and the Middle East, and if left untended can become impenetrable. The name derives from the leaves, which contain a milky sap and are recognizable by mottled splashes of white. Legend has it that milk fell from the Virgin Mary's breast onto the milk thistle plant as she fed baby Jesus, hence its folk names of Mary's Thistle, Our Lady's Thistle, and Holy Thistle.

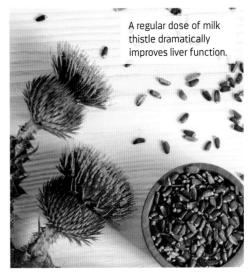

A regular dose of milk thistle dramatically improves liver function.

Those suffering from the previous night's excess will certainly feel that there's something holy about this thistle. It is probably most well known for its incredible liver-healing properties and has been used as a liver tonic for over 2,000 years. Milk thistle seeds contain the chemical compound silymarin, which has been shown to have dramatic healing effects on liver stresses ranging from cirrhosis of the liver and hepatitis to gallbladder disorders and patients undergoing chemotherapy. It is the liver that must deal with the onslaught of coffee, alcohol, drugs, fatty and junk foods, red meat, pesticides, and environmental pollutants that our bodies are often subjected to. This is where milk thistle comes into its own—a regular dose dramatically improves liver function.

Milk thistle has been used throughout history for medicinal healing.

Primitive negative emotions like anger are stored in the liver. Anger can be useful if it is used productively but it is often difficult to express anger in a healthy way. Sometimes we turn to addictions to block out real emotions. Milk thistle combined with meditation can help us to acknowledge and release anger.

It is thought that milk thistle found its way to Britain when the Roman armies arrived, taking the seeds, leaves, stalks, and roots with them to provide food and medicine. The Roman physician and naturalist Pliny the Elder wrote that the juice of the plant mixed with honey is excellent for "carrying off bile"—one of the earliest references to its liver-healing properties.

As its name suggests, milk thistle has been reported to be an effective aid to women who breastfeed, promoting milk flow. While there isn't clear evidence, a history of its use for such a reason is usually a pretty good indicator of its effectiveness. One of the huge benefits of this plant is that it is so safe and can be used by pregnant and breastfeeding women and children. Its detoxifying properties help with skin conditions such as acne, eczema, and psoriasis.

It is the black, shiny seeds that are used in most milk thistle preparations that can be purchased from health food shops. They were traditionally roasted and can be used as a coffee substitute. Although it is not so popular now, milk thistle used to be highly regarded as a food and was commonly grown in gardens for that purpose, the flower heads boiled and eaten like artichokes. The shoots are still popular in some countries today and are very palatable and nutritious, generally being cooked and eaten like cabbage. The leaves have a taste similar to spinach and can be used both as a cooked vegetable and as a delicious salad green.

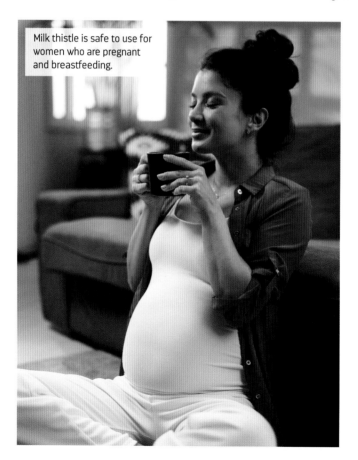

Milk thistle is safe to use for women who are pregnant and breastfeeding.

URINARY SYSTEM

THE HEALTH OF OUR KIDNEYS IS CRUCIAL TO OUR WELLBEING. THEY CARRY OUT the vital functions of preserving, cleaning, and circulating fluids in our bodies. Keeping our fluid levels balanced by drinking enough water and limiting the intake of dehydrating foods and drinks such as coffee and alcohol is essential. A lack of fluid in the body can lead to problems such as dry mouth, headaches, dry and itchy eyes, dry and clicky joints (due to a lack of synovial fluids), dry skin, and urinary tract problems.

Drinking the requisite half gallon (two liters) of fresh water a day is vital. As is reducing intake of sugary, fatty foods and trying to reintroduce more healthy, simple fare. Your body won't appreciate going cold turkey on all your usual treats, but you can simply add lots of greenery and whole grains to your diet to begin with. Gradually the body will detox, and you will find yourself reaching for more nourishing healthy foods. Pack in more dark-green vegetables, nuts, fruit, lean meat, and fish

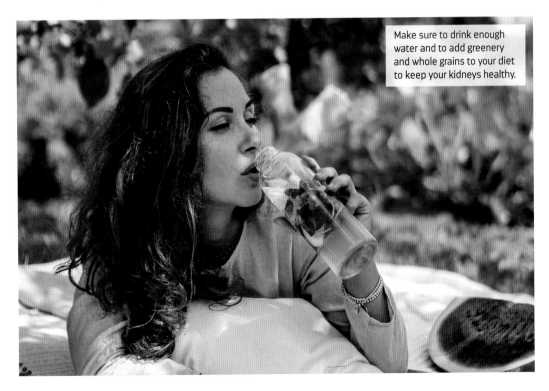

Make sure to drink enough water and to add greenery and whole grains to your diet to keep your kidneys healthy.

to keep your Vitamin B, iron, potassium, magnesium, copper, and zinc levels up; and broccoli, cabbage, oranges, and berries for Vitamin C.

Kidney imbalance leads to more than just feeling dehydrated. In Chinese medicine, the kidneys and bladder belong to the water element and the emotion related to this area is fear and anxiety. When the water element is balanced in our body and our kidneys are healthy, we have a healthy fear response; when it is out of balance, we either have no fear or we live in constant state of anxiety.

The main function of our kidneys is to remove toxins. The ancient practice of reflexology, which has been used for thousands of years to keep the body in balance, can help stimulate the kidneys and keep them in good working condition. Find the kidney points in the center of the feet. You can use your thumb to apply light pressure on this spot, using a small, circular movement to help boost your kidney function.

There are natural remedies that can be used to improve kidney function—celery seed and fennel are two key plants to use for the urinary system. You'll also be able to read about the incredible healing powers of urine on page 64. If you can get past the squeamishness, you'll discover a powerful healer available to you whenever you need it.

Kidney Stones

Kidney stones are a crystallization of the urine, often accompanied by pain and the passing of blood in the urine. Flush the kidneys with lemon juice taken in warm water three times a day. Use essential oil of lemon, fennel, and geranium in the bath or a few drops in a carrier oil, such as sweet almond oil, can be massaged into the lower back and bladder area. Make a tonic from celery seeds to benefit the kidneys.

Celery Seed Tonic

- 2 tablespoons celery seed
- 1 pint (600 ml) brandy
- 2 tablespoons water, for serving

1. Crush the celery seed in a pestle and mortar.

2. Place in a glass jar and cover with the brandy.

3. Leave for two weeks to infuse. Strain and store in a dark bottle.

4. Take 1 tablespoon daily mixed with water to boost kidney function

Urinary Complaints

Drink the water used to cook asparagus to treat general disorders of the urinary system.

Cystitis

Cystitis is an inflammation of the bladder, which causes burning pain when passing urine. The need to pee is frequent although often little, if any, urine is passed. Avoid scented bath products and drink plenty of water to flush the urinary system. Bio live yogurt can be applied to the vaginal area to encourage good bacteria. Oats are soothing to the system—see page 28 for a calming oat water tonic that can be taken regularly to help flush out the system and soothe inflammation caused by cystitis. Cantharis is the homeopathic remedy for treating cystitis. Cranberry juice or tea can be drunk to help flush out the system.

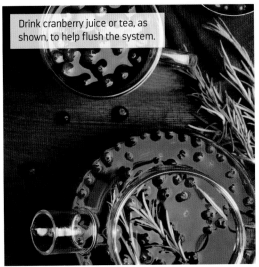

Drink cranberry juice or tea, as shown, to help flush the system.

Stress Incontinence

Stress incontinence is the uncontrollable passing of urine when there is pressure on the abdomen through laughing, sneezing, or after childbirth. Drink plenty of water to keep the bladder muscles working. Horsetail is a strengthening herb for the bladder. You can make this herb into a drink to aid bladder control.

Bladder-Strengthening Tea
- 1 teaspoon horsetail, chopped into small pieces
- 2 cups water

1. Place the horsetail in a saucepan.
2. Cover with the water and heat gently for thirty minutes.
3. Strain and drink a cup morning and night.

Urine Therapy

Your own urine has healing powers. Many people feel uneasy about using what they consider to be a waste product from the body as a therapeutic treatment and I must admit it took me several years to get over the "Urghh, why would anyone want to do that?" reaction that I had initially. Now that I have tried it on myself for several years and used it for my family too, I understand the healing properties of this gift from our bodies.

If you look at the ingredients on many skincare products, you'll often find urea listed. This is urine, often sourced from cattle, used for its skin-enhancing properties. Applying fresh urine to any cut, wound, burn, insect bite, or sting will help the body to heal. I have found it an incredible treatment for many skin problems and effective in treating aches and pains, too.

You can create a urine pack to treat areas of pain or discomfort in the body. When you have a headache for example, it is a good idea to place a urine pack on the liver region of the body (just under the ribs). Take a cloth and soak it in your own urine. Place the cloth over the area that you want to treat. Wrap a towel over the top around the body, followed by an old sheet. Place a shower curtain or plastic sheet on the bed and lie down with a hot water bottle on top of the wrapping that covers the urine pack. Rest for thirty minutes. You can use this as often as is required to relieve the pain. Urine is a quick-working therapy and many who have tried it see it as a miracle that we have such a strong and effective medicine available to us on tap and for free. Try it!

Plant Profile: Nettle

Stinging nettles (*urtica urens*) may not be an obvious choice for a useful and healing garden plant, but they offer many benefits to the gardener. They attract wildlife, can be woven into a strong hardwearing cloth, and have many healing properties. This plant can be found all over the temperate regions of the world and has much lore and legend attached to it. In Scandinavian mythology the nettle was sacred to Thor, God of Thunder. It was believed that if a plant was thrown onto a fire during a thunderstorm the house would be protected from lightning. Nettles were also thought to bring courage to the bearer and to drive away fearful thoughts in times of danger, so people often carried a small pouch of them if they were heading off on a long journey.

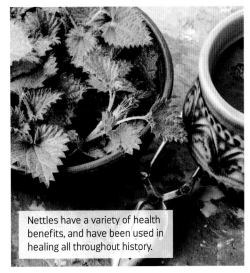

Nettles have a variety of health benefits, and have been used in healing all throughout history.

Romans reputedly planted nettles along the roadsides in Britain to warm themselves up. They thought that it would be so cold in Britain's chilly climes that they would need to thrash themselves with nettles to warm the blood. Native American Indians believed that the leaves held special powers and they were used in the treatment of aches and pains, while European herbalists were using the leaves in similar ways on the other side of the Atlantic to relieve gout and arthritis.

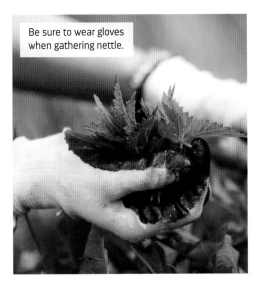

Be sure to wear gloves when gathering nettle.

An irritant found in the tiny hairs found on the leaf and stem—histamine—causes nettle's sting. Each hair is hollow with the venom stored at its base. When the hair is brushed against, it breaks off exposing a sharp point which penetrates the skin and delivers the sting. How wonderfully clever nature is to invent such a complex weapon against predators and then to counteract this with an offering of dock leaves, which can usually be found growing nearby. The leaves of dock, when rubbed on the affected area, release a chemical that neutralizes the sting and soothes the skin.

Nettles have long been used as food and even Pepys wrote of eating ". . . some nettle porridge, which was very good." This plant is an excellent source of calcium, iron, magnesium, and a range of vitamins. Young nettles can be gathered (while wearing gloves) and steeped in a pot of boiling water to create an excellent spring tonic, which helps to clear out the toxins accumulated during the winter months. When dried or cooked, the nettle loses its sting. Nettle tea has many beneficial uses, such as treatment of rheumatism and urinary disorders and it is also a rich source of iron and calcium for pregnant women. It can be used to good effect after birth too as it stimulates milk flow in lactating mothers. Nettle tea has also been shown to be beneficial in treating skin rashes.

Soothing Nettle Tea

Drink regularly to boost calcium, iron, and magnesium levels. Be sure to wear gloves when harvesting and pick out the top four leaves before the plant flowers (early spring and autumn).

- 1 handful fresh nettle tops (or 1 tablespoon dried nettle leaves)
- 1 cup water, just off the boil

1. Place the nettle tops or dried leaves into a cup.

2. Pour the water on top.

3. Cover and leave to steep for ten minutes.

4. Strain and enjoy up to three cups a day.

To get a nettle patch started in your garden, look for a sunny sheltered spot and ensure that the soil is well nourished. Find a friend who can donate some plants for your plot—an allotment owner or keen gardener should be only too happy to give you some. Nettles are wild so should not be taken from the countryside. Plant the nettles about 11¾ inches (30 cm) apart and keep them well watered. It is a good idea to fix a path or boundary around your patch as nettles can quickly take over. Then sit back and watch your garden thrive and your health blossom as you use this powerful cleansing, balancing plant.

Respiratory System

RESPIRATORY PROBLEMS OF ALL KINDS CAN RESPOND WELL TO ALTERNATIVE therapies. The two most common problems affecting the nose are the common cold and hay fever. Colds can be treated very effectively with herbs—there are several decongestant plants that can be used. Sometimes on an unconscious level when we are disappointed or disillusioned, we develop colds and sinus problems. The nose being blocked can represent a holding on to tears due to holding on to grief or disappointment.

The remedies in this section can help balance the emotions and unblock the nose. You'll find out how to make a peppermint steam bath to clear the nasal passages and find ways of treating build-up of catarrh and sinusitis. For hay fever, the traditional remedy is a teaspoon of local honey taken every morning upon waking before the season begins. Elderflower is also a very effective remedy, and you'll find a recipe that you can use to make your own tea, which can be taken internally to lessen the severity of your symptoms.

Use natural healing to cleanse your respiratory system and feel better than ever.

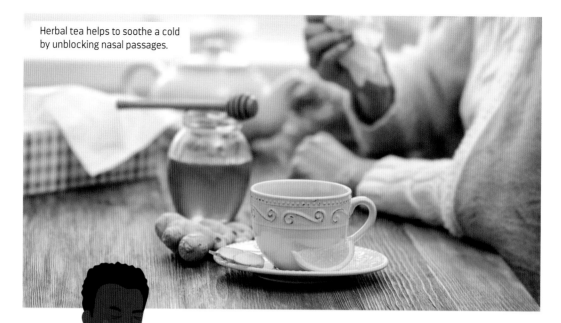

Herbal tea helps to soothe a cold by unblocking nasal passages.

Flu

The flu is a viral disease of the upper respiratory tract resulting in fever, aching limbs, runny nose, sore throat, and sometimes nausea and loss of appetite. It is important to allow the body to rest completely and to keep fluid levels up. Barley water can be used to treat respiratory disorders and is also useful in easing a dry tickly cough.

Barley Water

- 2 tablespoons barley
- 5 cups (1,200 ml) water, divided

1. Add barley to water. Boil for ten minutes.
2. Strain through a muslin cloth and add the barley to a fresh pint of water.
3. Boil this batch for ten minutes.
4. Strain and drink warm or cold, as often as required. Add lemon and honey to taste, as desired.

Hay Fever

Hay fever is an allergic reaction to airborne irritants like pollen. Swelling of the nasal passages accompanies red itchy eyes. Symptoms include sneezing and a runny nose. Lots of sufferers use local honey to treat hay fever. Take a teaspoon every day to ease symptoms. Eyebright tea can be used to soothe itchy eyes. Make an elderflower tea that can be taken internally to strengthen the immune system and help to prevent hay fever. The flowers can also be enjoyed fresh to relieve the symptoms.

Elderflower Tea

- 1 handful elderflower flowers
- Boiling water, as needed

1. Place elderflowers in a cup. Cover with boiling water.
2. Place a plate over the cup and leave to infuse for ten minutes.
3. Drink while still warm, up to three cups a day.

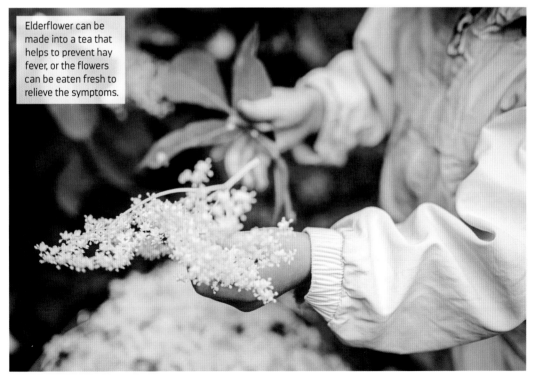

Elderflower can be made into a tea that helps to prevent hay fever, or the flowers can be eaten fresh to relieve the symptoms.

Common Cold

The common cold is an infection of the upper respiratory tract, which is very common, especially during the winter months. Excess mucus is produced, and the usual symptoms are a runny nose, sore throat, and coughing. Colds can also produce a fever, which is the body's natural way of fighting an infection. Work with the body rather than against it when a fever sets in. The most important thing to remember is the body's need for rest when an infection like a cold takes over.

If you do not allow yourself to deal with the infection naturally, if you suppress it with painkillers or decongestant drugs, then you will just be burying the problem and it will crop up again later as you won't have given your body a chance to remove unwanted toxins from the system. The quickest method for treating a cold is to make a honey and lemon tea. You can also make a honey and onion syrup to treat coughs and colds. **Note: if your fever lasts longer than three to five days or if it reaches 103°F (39.4°C) or higher, seek medical attention.**

Quick-Healing Tea

Try this super effective healing remedy for treatment of colds and cough.

- Juice of ½ lemon
- 1 tablespoon local honey
- 1-inch knob of ginger root, sliced
- 1 cup boiling water

1. Place the lemon juice, honey, and ginger root into a cup of boiling water.

2. Cover and allow to steep for ten minutes.

3. Drink warm. Enjoy often throughout the day to soothe symptoms and boost the respiratory system.

Honey and Onion Syrup

- 1 onion, sliced
- Honey, as needed

1. Lay the sliced onion in a shallow bowl. Cover with honey and leave overnight.

2. In the morning, pour off the liquid and use as needed. 1 tablespoon can be taken three times a day to treat a common cold.

Sinusitis

Sinusitis is the inflammation of the sinuses—the air-filled cavities around the nose—that causes a blocked, uncomfortable feeling. A peppermint steam bath can be beneficial to help release the blockage. You can also try this with essential oil of lavender, eucalyptus, and tea tree. Lavender acts as an anti-inflammatory and will ease any pain. Elderflower is the plant traditionally used to treat sinusitis. You can make a nose wash using the flowers, which grace the hedgerows in late spring.

Elderflower Nasal Wash

- 2 sprigs elderflower
- Boiling water, as needed
- Pinch salt

1. Place the elderflowers in a cup. Cover with boiling water and allow to cool slightly.

2. Add the salt.

3. Take the cup to the nose and sniff through each nostril in turn. This can be practiced morning and evening to relieve symptoms.

Peppermint Steam Bath

- 1 handful fresh peppermint leaves
- Boiling water, as needed

1. Cover peppermint leaves with boiling water.

2. Place a towel over your head.

3. Lean over the bowl and inhale the steam from the peppermint.

Nosebleeds

Nosebleeds are sometimes caused by infection of the mucus membrane. Massage a drop of lavender into the nostril to help the area to heal and to stop the flow of blood. Lean forward and lightly pinch the bridge of the nose to ease the flow. Take rescue remedy in cases of emotional distress.

Hot honey and lemon tea soothes a sore throat fast.

Sore Throat

A sore throat is inflammation of the throat caused by infection. Pain with difficulty in swallowing, sometimes accompanied by a fever, earache, and hoarseness. Lymph nodes in the neck become enlarged and tender. Gargle with honey water to soothe the throat. Add 1 tablespoon of honey to a cup of warm water, stir to dissolve, and then gargle with the liquid. Drink a hot honey and lemon tea recipe on page 70) before bed to ease symptoms and encourage a restful night's sleep.

Apple Cider Vinegar Compress

Apply an apple cider vinegar compress to the throat area to ease a sore throat.

- ½ cup apple cider vinegar (see page 109)
- Boiling water, as needed

1. Pour the apple cider vinegar into a large bowl. Top up with boiling water.
2. Leave to infuse for ten minutes.
3. Soak a cloth in the liquid, wring out, and apply to the throat area.
4. Lie down and relax for fifteen minutes with the compress on the throat.

Cough

Coughing is an action taken by the body to remove foreign bodies and mucus from the airways. Make a garlic tincture to treat coughs. This will help the body fight infection.

Garlic Tincture

- 5 garlic cloves, peeled
- Organic vodka or brandy, as needed

1. Place the garlic cloves in a glass jar. Cover with the alcohol and seal.

2. Leave to infuse for two weeks.

3. Strain and take a teaspoon as required to ease a cough. Can be taken up to three times a day.

Asthma

Asthma is inflammation of the lining of the airways, which results in restriction of airflow and breathing difficulty. Make a steam inhalation of lavender, chamomile, or eucalyptus to help open the airways. (Recipe on page 74.) Take a few drops of rescue remedy on the tongue at the start of an attack to help lessen the effects.

Pneumonia

Pneumonia is an infection of the lung caused by bacteria or virus entering the upper respiratory tract. This results in inflammation of the lung tissue. Rapid shallow breathing, chest pain, sore throat, and fever accompany. Raw garlic in the diet will help aid the body in fighting the infection. To help ease the breathing, make a steam bath using eucalyptus and tea tree essential oils. (Recipe on page 74.)

Healing Steam Bath

Help open the airways with a soothing steam bath. Use different essential oils as needed. Chamomile is soothing and calming, lavender antiseptic and calming, eucalyptus clearing, tea tree cleansing.

- 1 large bowl boiling water
- 2 drops each of eucalyptus and tea tree essential oils
- 1 large towel

1. Add the essential oils to the boiling water.

2. Create a tent over the bowl with the towel.

3. Put your head inside the tent, over the bowl, and inhale the cleansing system.

Lung Infection/Bronchitis

This is the inflammation of the lining of the air tubes of the lungs. Can cause chest pain, fever, wheezing, and shortness of breath and a hacking cough. Licorice root is beneficial in the treatment of bronchitis. Lung disorders can be treated with garlic syrup.

Garlic Syrup

- 8 cloves garlic, peeled and crushed
- 10 tablespoons honey

1. Place the crushed garlic in a glass jar and cover with the honey.

2. Allow to stand for several days.

3. Use as needed (1 teaspoon for children, 4 teaspoons for adults, twice daily).

Catarrh

Catarrh, an overproduction of thick phlegm by the mucus membranes, is often the result of a heavy cold. Many aromatherapy oils are decongestants. Make a blend using chamomile, pine, or clary sage. Rub this into the temples. You can also use these oils in a steam bath. Take a large bowl, fill with boiling water, add a few drops of your chosen oil, lean over, and inhale the steam. Make a mustard footbath to warm the body and help to decongest the nasal passages.

Decongestant Temple Rub

Use this as needed to soothe sinus pains and relieve congestion. Choose chamomile for soothing, pine for clearing, and clary sage for uplifting.

- 1 cup carrier oil, such as sweet almond
- 2 drops essential oil (either chamomile, pine, or clary sage)

Mix the oils together and rub into temples as needed.

Mustard Footbath

- Hot water, as needed
- 1 teaspoon mustard powder

1. Fill a washing bowl with hot water.
2. Add mustard powder and stir to disperse.
3. Place feet in the bowl and stay for fifteen minutes or until water starts to cool.

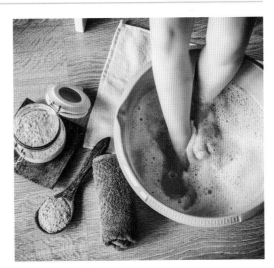

Plant Profile: Lavender

Lavender is an evergreen woody shrub, which grows up to 1 yard (1 meter) tall, with pale-green, narrow leaves and flowers of a beautiful violet/blue color. It has an immediately recognizable scent when you gently press the flower spike between your finger and thumb. Endowed with both antiseptic and sedative properties, lavender's supreme versatility has led some to call it nature's medicine chest. Almost everyone is familiar with the smell of the lavender plant, and it has over 2,500 years of recorded use as a strewing herb, a mood tonic, a fragrance, an insect repellent, a medicine, and a food flavoring. The twenty-eight different species of lavender are grown for their flowers and for their essential oil.

In ancient times lavender was used for mummification and perfume by the Egyptians, Phoenicians, and peoples of Arabia. The Greeks and the Romans bathed in lavender-scented water, and it was from the Latin word *lavo* meaning "to wash" that the herb took its name. Lavender has long been used to clean and heal wounds—the Romans used it for this purpose and in more recent history, nurses used it for the wounded soldiers during WWII.

Lavender has many royal connections. Queen Elizabeth I valued lavender as a conserve and a perfume. Her love of lavender was such that she is supposed to have commanded her gardeners to ensure that fresh lavender flowers should be available all year round. She also used lavender infused in hot water to make a tea to help ease her migraines. Queen Victoria also had a passion for this plant and is responsible for making lavender popular as a perfume. She used it in every one of her rooms, for washing floors and furniture, freshening the air, and for scattering amongst the linens.

Lavender has been used for over 2,500 years for medicinal, fragrant, and culinary use.

The seventeenth-century medical herbalist Nicholas Culpeper recommended this plant for a variety of ailments, including pains of the head, cramps, and fainting. Lavender is one of the main essential oils. It is an invaluable oil to have around the house for any number of little, and large, emergencies. The oil can be dabbed neat (without dilution in a base oil) onto the skin immediately after burning to speed up the skin's healing processes, and for this reason alone it is an essential part of any home first aid kit. The essential oil of lavender can also be used to ease stress and anxiety and is best used in a burner or vaporizer to promote a calm and peaceful environment.

For colds, flu, and catarrh, try adding two drops of lavender oil to a bowl of boiled water and putting your head over the steam for about five minutes to inhale the healing properties. One of the most soothing uses for lavender is in a hot compress for period and labor pains, arthritis, and headaches.

Hot Compress for Period Pains

Can also be used to treat arthritis, labor pains, and headaches.

- 1 bowl hot water
- 6 drops lavender essential oil
- Flannel or facecloth

1. Add lavender oil into the bowl.
2. Soak the cloth in the hot water, squeeze out excess liquid, and place over the affected area until the cloth cools.
3. Repeat as needed.

A cold compress is another way to reap the benefits of lavender and more useful for sprains, burns and scalds, insect bites, stings, and sunburn. A cool flannel infused with lavender is a great comfort when your skin is taut and painful after overexposure to the sun.

Cool Compress for Sunburn

Can also be used to treat insect bites and stings.

- 1 bowl of cold water
- 6 drops of lavender essential oil
- Flannel or facecloth

1. Add lavender oil to the bowl.
2. Soak the cloth in cool water, squeeze out excess liquid, and place over the affected area.
3. Repeat as needed.

Lavender is also one of the few oils that can be used neat on the skin. It can be dabbed directly onto spots, boils, cuts, grazes, burns, insect bites, acne, and other skin conditions. A few drops on a handkerchief or tissue can be used to calm symptoms of sudden stress, panic, hysteria, shock, and butterflies in the stomach.

You can grow your own lavender plants for use in food and for potpourri and linen. The tender varieties such as French and Spanish lavender can be grown outside in pots in summer, then brought inside to a bright windowsill for the winter. The soil in the pot should contain some sand to aid drainage. While these varieties are not as fragrant as the hardy lavenders, they will reward you with blooms almost all year round. Harvest lavender for drying when the first bud on the flower stalk is starting to open. To dry, bind stems with a rubber band or string and hang in a warm, dry, dark spot. When dry, pack away in boxes or plastic bags for medicinal or culinary use.

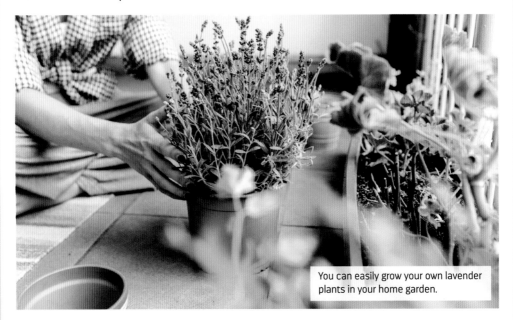

You can easily grow your own lavender plants in your home garden.

THE SKIN

OUR SKIN IS THE ORGAN MOST IN TOUCH WITH THE OUTSIDE WORLD. IT protects us from our environment, releases toxins, and keeps our body temperature in balance by opening and closing pores and releasing sweat to cool the body.

Spots, sweating, hair loss, and rashes are usually symptoms of other, deeper-seated problems—for example, acne is often caused by a hormone imbalance. Sweating disorders include a lack of sweating or excess sweating. In traditional Chinese medicine, excess heat in the body can lead to dryness, itching, redness, and flaking of skin cells. Cooling herbs and foods such as cucumber and mint can be taken regularly to balance the body temperature.

The skin is the largest organ of the body. The bowels excrete waste, the kidneys excrete fluids, lungs excrete gases, and skin excretes anything else. Therefore, skin symptoms present when there

Cooling foods like cucumber balance the body temperature and hydrate skin.

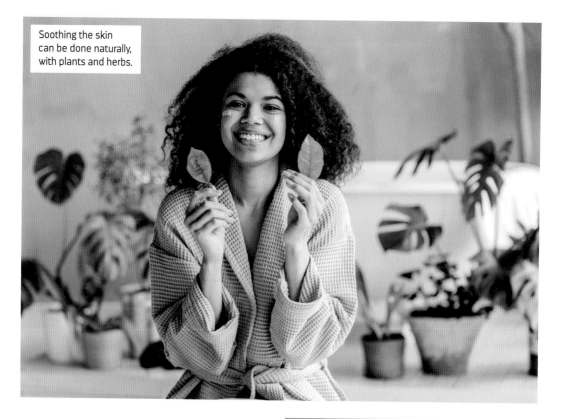

Soothing the skin can be done naturally, with plants and herbs.

is an imbalance in the body. Eczema, psoriasis, and other skin conditions often result when the other elimination channels are blocked.

Skin rashes can be an allergic reaction to an outside agent (such as perfumed soap, deodorants, washing powders, textiles, or metals in clothing); they can result from foods or medications or drugs, or be a reaction to something the body does not tolerate. In this chapter you can find out how to make your own deodorant to treat excess perspiration, try a soothing oatmeal bath to ease the symptoms of eczema, and use plantain to heal insect bites and stings.

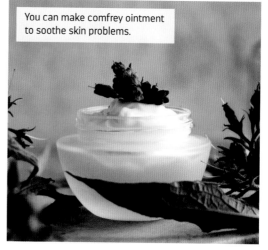

You can make comfrey ointment to soothe skin problems.

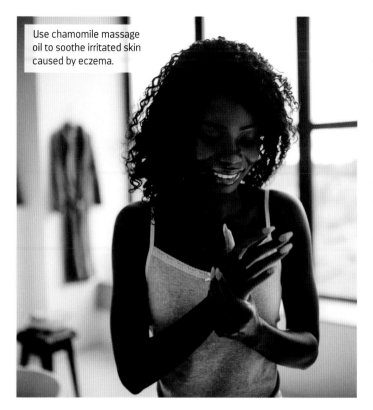
Use chamomile massage oil to soothe irritated skin caused by eczema.

Eczema

This is a skin inflammation that is visible through red cracked patches of skin, common on hands, feet, and behind the ears. The symptoms are burning, itching skin with a desire to scratch. Sometimes the skin blisters can open and weep. See page 149 for advice on how to treat children's eczema. The essential oil chamomile can be very soothing to irritated skin. Oats can be used to make a soothing bath treatment, which calms red, itchy skin and is beneficial before bed to help aid a restful night's sleep.

Chamomile Massage Oil

Use to soothe irritated skin. Try a patch test first in case of sensitivity.

- 4 ounces organic olive oil
- 2 drops chamomile essential oil

1. Add the chamomile to the carrier oil.
2. Massage into affected areas to soothe dry skin and irritation.

Oatmeal Bath

- 1 handful oats

1. Take oats and place in the center of a square of muslin cloth.
2. Gather the oats in the cloth. Secure with a piece of string or a rubber band.
3. Place in a warm bath and enjoy.

Incorporate more raw garlic into your diet to help combat the effects of psoriasis on the skin.

Psoriasis

A skin disorder that tends to run in families, psoriasis presents as patches of red skin with a scaly silvery surface. Often affects the armpits and insides of the knees and elbows. There are ways to treat the irritated skin with natural remedies but as with all skin disorders, psoriasis is symptomatic of an imbalance in the body so it is worth looking at what this might be. Does the condition flare up at times of stress or when you eat certain foods, for example? If you can identify the trigger, it will help you to address the problem holistically. Use the cleansing powers of garlic by including more of it in your diet. It is particularly beneficial eaten raw, so grate into salads or soups just before serving. Nettle tea helps to cleanse the system and is especially useful in the spring and early summer.

Prickly Heat

Prickly heat is a heat rash that occurs in particularly hot and humid weather. Chickweed ointment can be massaged into the affected area and helps to calm irritated skin. A massage with organic sweet almond oil combined with a few drops of lavender can be a beneficial treatment.

Perspiration

Excessive sweating is usually caused by the body's need to regulate temperature. Commercial antiperspirants work by blocking the sweat ducts under your armpits. Sweat is your body's way of removing toxins from the body, so daily blocking of this simple and effective strategy is not ideal and can cause longer-term health problems. It is bacteria mixing with your sweat, rather than the sweat itself, that causes body odor and these deodorants will only work to mask this smell.

Baking soda works wonders as deodorant as it neutralizes the odor of sweat. Just sprinkle a light covering onto a damp flannel and pat on. There is no need to rinse.

Deodorant Powder

- 8 tablespoons baking soda
- 8 tablespoons cornstarch
- A few drops lavender or lemon essential oils

1. Place the baking soda, cornstarch, and essential oils in a glass jar.
2. Shake to blend.
3. Sprinkle a light covering of the powder onto a flannel and pat on. Do not rinse.

Liquid Deodorant

- 4 tablespoons witch hazel extract
- 4 tablespoons aloe vera gel
- 4 tablespoons mineral water
- 1 teaspoon vegetable glycerin
- A few drops lavender or tea tree essential oils

1. Put all the ingredients in a spray bottle and shake to blend.
2. Spray on as needed.

Comfrey ointment can reduce acne scarring.

Acne

Our skin has sebaceous glands that secret an oily substance. Sometimes these glands get overactive and secrete excessive oil and that causes acne. Prepare a facial steam bath to draw out infection. Comfrey ointment can be used to reduce acne scarring.

Comfrey Ointment

- 1¼ pounds (500 g) beeswax
- 2¼ ounces (60 g) dried or 5 ounces (150 g) fresh comfrey leaves, finely chopped

1. Melt the beeswax in a glass bowl over a pan of boiling water.
2. Add the comfrey leaves and simmer, stirring continuously, for about one hour.
3. Pour the mixture into a muslin bag.
4. Wearing rubber gloves, squeeze the mixture through the bag into a jug.
5. Pour the ointment into a jar before it sets. Place the lid on the jar, without securing it.
6. When cool, tighten the lid. Store in a refrigerator for up to three months.

Facial Steam Bath

- 1 handful chickweed flowers
- 1 handful elderflower flowers
- 1 handful calendula flowers
- Hot water, as needed

1. Fill a bowl with hot water and add the flowers.
2. Place a towel over your head and inhale the steam for ten minutes.
3. Repeat daily to improve the health of your skin.

Athlete's Foot

Athlete's foot is a fungal infection that grows in the warm, moist skin between the toes. Apply a garlic poultice directly to the affected area. Crush two cloves of garlic, place on the foot, and secure with a plaster. Leave on for as long as possible, up to one hour. Make a footbath using essential oils with anti-fungal properties.

Anti-Fungal Footbath

- A few drops lavender essential oil
- A few drops tea tree essential oil
- A few drops patchouli essential oil
- Hot water, as needed

1. Fill a large bowl with the hot water and add the essential oils.
2. Place your feet in the bowl and relax for fifteen minutes.

Chilblains

This is circular red swelling that usually appears on the toes, but can affect the hands too, during cold weather. Caused by poor circulation, or the narrowing of the arteries in cold conditions, restricting the flow of blood. Encourage the circulatory system by drinking warming teas such as ginger and rosemary. Make a poultice out of crushed horseradish root and apply to the affected area to encourage healing.

Horseradish Poultice

As well as treating chilblains, this poultice can be used to ease joint and muscle pain.

- 2 tablespoons horseradish root, grated
- Large cloth

1. Place grated horseradish onto cloth.
2. Tie at the top and place directly onto affected area.

Cuts and Sores

When the surface of the skin is damaged it can result in an infection, and the surrounding area becomes red and sore. Make a poultice of cabbage leaves to draw out the infection and aid healing. Yarrow is also very beneficial in the treatment of cuts and sores. Make your own yarrow tincture, which can be diluted one part to ten parts water. Soak a cloth in the liquid and bathe the wound with it.

Cabbage Poultice

This has an anti-inflammatory effect and can be used for swollen joints or to ease bruising. Also try for sore throats and to treat mastitis when breastfeeding.

- Several cabbage leaves
- Pan of boiling water

1. Crush the cabbage leaves, gently with a rolling pin. Pop into a pan of boiling water for a few minutes.
2. Wrap the warm leaves around the affected area. Leave on for up to a couple hours.
3. Hold in place with clothing or saran wrap.

Yarrow Tincture

- Flowering tops of yarrow plant, as needed
- Alcohol such as organic vodka, as needed

1. Pick the flowering tops of the yarrow plant, white ones only, when in bloom.
2. Fill, but don't stuff, a jar with the coarsely chopped herb.
3. Fill jar to the top with the alcohol.
4. Cap tightly. The yarrow tincture will be ready to use in six weeks.

Cold Sores

Cold sores are fluid-filled blisters caused by a viral infection (herpes simplex). They usually appear around the mouth, on the lips, or under the nose. They are very contagious and can be painful. Often a symptom of high levels of stress or feeling run down. As soon as it appears, apply St. John's Wort tincture to the cold sore. Place a few drops of lemon juice on the core sore every day until it goes. Lemons have antiseptic and anti-fungal properties.

St John's Wort Tincture

- 1 handful flowering tops from the St. John's Wort plant
- 7 fluid ounces (200 ml) alcohol, such as vodka
- 3½ fluid ounces (100 ml) water

1. Place the flowering tops in a large glass jar.
2. Cover with the alcohol and water.
3. Replace the lid and leave for two weeks, shaking occasionally.
4. Strain through a sieve with a muslin cloth inside.
5. Pour the liquid into a clean dark glass bottle and store for up to one year.

Sunstroke

Sunstroke occurs when the body becomes overheated through overexposure to the sun and the brain cannot control the cooling process. Sunstroke is different from and more dangerous than heat stroke. Both conditions cause confusion, lightheadedness, and fatigue. Shade and cool water on the skin helps. Peppermint has a cooling, soothing effect when taken internally. Drink a cooling tea to help your body get back to its regular temperature. **Note: if you are still experiencing extreme heat after thirty minutes of using these methods, you should seek medical attention.**

Cooling Tea

- 1 handful peppermint leaves
- Boiling water, as needed
- Juice of ½ lemon

1. Place the peppermint leaves in a cup and cover with boiling water.
2. Allow to cool.
3. Add the lemon juice and place in refrigerator. When ready to drink, add ice.

You can place plantain directly on skin, as shown here, or use the leaf to make a soothing lotion.

Rashes

A rash is a red eruption of the skin that changes the way the skin looks and feels. Rashes can be localized to one area or may be widespread. Plantain is a wonder plant when it comes to skin problems. Apply this soothing lotion to areas of irritable skin and to treat rashes.

Healing Skin Lotion

- 2 handfuls plantain leaves
- Glycerin, as needed

1. Take the plantain leaves and crush in a pestle with a mortar.

2. Place in a glass jar and add the glycerin (available from chemists) to cover the leaves.

3. Leave for two weeks, stirring occasionally.

4. Strain and store in a dark glass bottle.

5. Use as needed to treat irritable skin conditions.

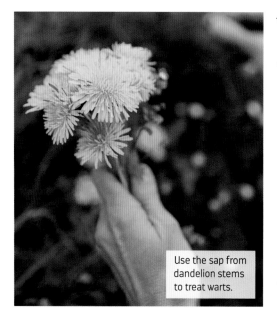

Use the sap from dandelion stems to treat warts.

Warts

A hard, raised growth on the skin is referred to as a wart. Warts come in various sizes and shapes and they can affect any age group. They usually grow to certain size and then stop. They commonly appear on the neck, fingers, face, scalp, and pretty much any other part of the skin. They sometimes disappear on their own but rubbing freshly squeezed lemon juice into the skin every day can aid the healing process. Eat plenty of garlic and apply a slice of cut garlic to the wart in the evening, secured with a plaster or piece of cloth wrapped and tied around to keep it secure. Use the sap from a dandelion plant to remove warts. Squeeze the milky sap from the stem of a large leaf. Apply once a day until the wart heals.

Boils

An infected hair follicle with a swollen pus-filled area is called a boil. A painful red lump later becomes a yellow-headed spot. Most commonly occurring under the arms, back of the neck, and in the groin. Make a boil treatment using thyme leaves, soak a cloth in it, and apply to the boil.

Boil Treatment

- 1 handful thyme leaves
- Boiling water, as needed

1. Place the thyme leaves in a cup. Cover with boiling water and allow to steep for ten minutes.
2. Soak a cloth in the liquid and apply to the affected area.

Massage rosemary essential oil into your scalp to stimulate hair growth.

Hair Loss

We shed 150 hairs a day, but this number can be increased by stress. Rosemary is a traditional hair tonic. Massage a few drops of rosemary essential oil into the scalp. It is said that the increased flow of blood to the head in positions such as shoulder stand in yoga can have a beneficial effect on hair growth. You can even reap the benefits during a supported leg raise. Find a wall with no obstructions and lie on your back with your legs raised at right angles up the wall. Drink a regular cup of sage tea to stimulate hair growth.

Sage Tea

- 1 handful sage leaves
- Boiling water, as needed

1. Place the sage leaves in a cup.
2. Cover with boiling water, place a plate over the top, and leave to infuse for ten minutes.
3. Drink a cup every morning—up to three cups a day.

Dandruff

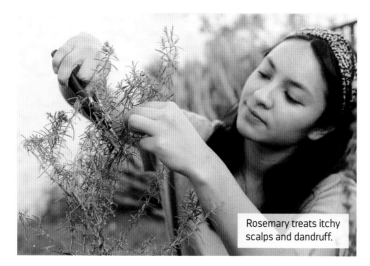

Rosemary treats itchy scalps and dandruff.

When the scalp sheds dead skin cells in large clumps, the flakes can get trapped in the hair and accumulate with oil and dirt to cause dandruff. Scaling may be accompanied by mild itching, causing redness and flaking. Dandruff can also occur in the eyebrows. Rosemary is the traditional treatment for itchy, irritable scalps and dandruff.

Rosemary Vinegar

- 1 ounce (25 g) fresh rosemary, chopped
- 2 pints (1.2 liters) cider vinegar

1. Place the rosemary in a large glass jar and cover with the cider vinegar.

2. Leave for two weeks, shaking occasionally.

3. Strain and bottle the liquid.

4. Massage 2 tablespoons into the hair, half an hour before washing.

Sunburn

Spending too long in the sun can cause the skin to burn. It feels hot, tingly, and uncomfortable and becomes red and hot to the touch. Calendula oil is soothing to the system and helps the skin to heal effectively and prevent scarring. (Recipe on opposite page.) Take a cool bath, gently massage the oil into the affected areas, and then rest.

Calendula Oil

- 1 handful dried calendula flowers
- Sweet almond oil or apricot kernel oil, as needed

1. Place the dried flowers in a glass jar with a lid and cover completely with the oil.

2. Seal tightly and leave to infuse for three to eight weeks, shaking daily.

3. When the oil has turned golden, strain through a piece of muslin and bottle it in a dark glass bottle. Store in the refrigerator and use to treat skin conditions such as wounds, pimples, and sunburn.

Insect Bites

These are very common from late spring through to autumn. Use a burner to diffuse essential oil of citronella on summer evenings or use citronella candles. Some people find that eating plenty of garlic keeps the mosquitoes away. You can also rub lemon juice, a natural insecticide, into the skin to discourage mosquitos and other small biting insects.

Once bitten, to help calm itchy, irritated skin, apply plantain oil topically. Plantain starts to come into leaf mid spring, so it is perfect timing to get a batch of oil started ready for the hotter months when biting insects are more prevalent.

Plantain Oil

Choose a dry, sunny day and harvest the plantain in the afternoon (once the dew has dried).

- Plantain leaves, as needed
- Olive oil, as needed

1. Tightly pack a clean, dry jar full of plantain leaves and fill with olive oil.

2. Place the jar out of direct sunlight and store at room temperature for three weeks, topping the oil up so that it completely covers the leaves every day for the first week.

3. Strain the oil and apply to itchy, irritated skin.

Plant Profile: Calendula

Also known as the Pot Marigold, *Calendula officinalis* is an easy-to-grow plant, which has numerous uses and healing properties. The vibrant orange-and-yellow flowers are said to lift the spirits and encourage cheerfulness. However, this colorful flowering plant is perhaps best known for its skin-healing properties. It can be used to treat wounds, burns, insect bites, eczema, skin ulcers, and rashes. Indeed, many herbalists use calendula in their preparations, and arthroscopic medicinal producer Weleda have a special range of soothing calendula products. An infusion of the petals can be used for flu and fevers as it helps to induce perspiration. For ear infections, a drop of oil on a cotton ball can be effective. The soothing properties of calendula can also be useful to treat sore nipples and diaper rash.

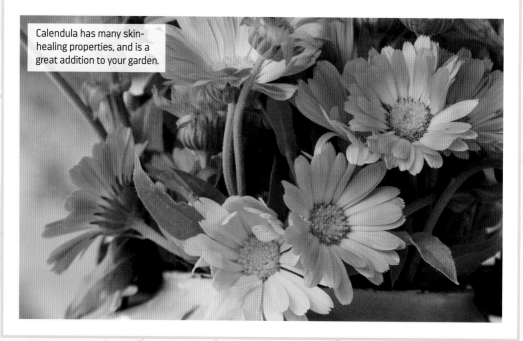

Calendula has many skin-healing properties, and is a great addition to your garden.

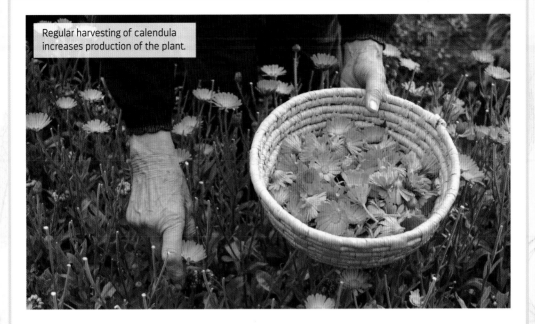
Regular harvesting of calendula increases production of the plant.

The plant is grown easily from seed in spring and while calendula prefers rich well-drained soil, it is very tolerant of poor soils. Choose a sunny spot and you can enjoy the pleasure of growing your own medicine. As the plant flowers, pinch the heads and leave these to dry in a cool place out of direct sunlight and free from moisture. Regular harvesting of the flowers increases production. Store the dried flower heads in jars and use as needed. Be sure to leave some flower heads at the end of the flowering season so that you can collect the seeds and start afresh next year.

It is thought that the calendula plant originated in the Mediterranean and North Africa, and it was certainly valued highly by the Ancient Egyptians and Romans when it was known as the "Herb of the Sun". In Christianity, the flower was associated with the Virgin Mary, from which the common name Marigold (Mary Gold) is derived. In addition to healing humans, Calendula has also been used to treat animals for centuries. Three handfuls of flowers mixed with their food twice daily is said to aid heart problems, vomiting, and skin conditions. A lotion can be made to treat bee and wasp stings by boiling chopped leaves and flowers in milk.

The petals of calendula flowers have long been used to flavor foods. When fresh they have a very mild flavor but once cooked impart a savory taste, which complements soups, stews, and baked foods like bread and scones. In the summer, the flower heads make a beautiful addition to salads. A preserve can be made by placing whole leaves and petals in a wide-mouthed jar. Cover with sugar and leave until a syrup forms. Fresh calendula flowers heighten the energy in a room and have been used to attract and see fairies! Placed under a pillow before bed, the flowers apparently encourage clairvoyancy and petals scattered under the bed protect you in your sleep and make your dreams come true. Calendula is a truly magical, bright flower that deserves a sunny spot in your garden.

HEART AND BLOOD HEALTH

IT'S IMPORTANT FOR BOTH MEN AND WOMEN TO TAKE CARE OF THEIR HEART and blood health. Exercise is a great way to start.

Heart attack rates are increasing, with significantly higher rates for men. The typical causes are smoking, high cholesterol, high blood pressure, and obesity, all of which are as prevalent in women as they are in men. So why the gender divide?

One theory is that men need to change the way that they deal with emotions to start healing their hearts. The heart is incredibly sensitive to stress, and many systems of medicine recommend that we regularly take notice of the feelings and functions of the heart and care for this strong but sensitive muscle.

This school of thought believes that the emotional reserve of many men begins in childhood when they receive less physical affection and hugging than their female siblings. The giving and receiving of affection in the form of touch and embrace conveys positive emotions and nourishes the heart. Perhaps if men were encouraged to express their emotions more readily heart disease would be less prevalent. Tears should be allowed to flow freely to express feelings of happiness and experiences of

It's important for both men and women to take care of their heart and blood health. Exercise is a great way to start.

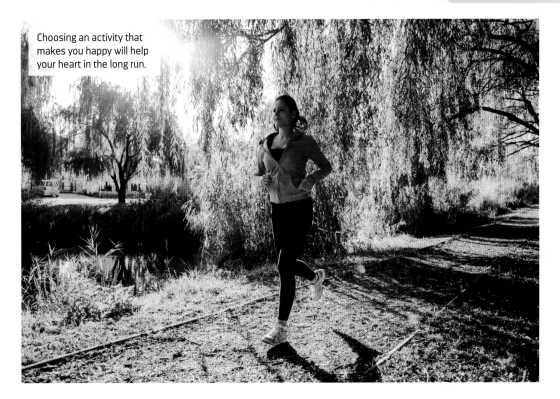

Choosing an activity that makes you happy will help your heart in the long run.

frustration, grief, and pain. If we can begin to see crying as a healthy response to life, it will help us to rid the body's build-up of stress. Suppressing tears is likely to increase the body's susceptibility to illness and blocking emotions can contribute to hypertension or high blood pressure.

Nourishing the Heart

Get in balance: Express yourself—both the positive and the negative feelings and emotions.

Laugh and play: Balance productivity with playfulness. Scientific studies have shown that laughter boosts the immune system by replacing hormones that act as immune suppressants.

Keep fit: Exercise develops the muscles and provides the rhythmic contraction and relaxation of the skeletal muscles that help circulate blood.

Eat simply: Eat whole grains, vegetables, and organic proteins. Avoid excess salt, sugar, additives, and processed good.

Use herbs: Plants that are especially good for the heart muscle are hawthorn, motherwort, yarrow, garlic, ginger, and cayenne.

Of course, a strong heart is necessary to keep limbs and organs in shape, and, equally, to help us cope with life's ups and downs. The way we use or abuse it has serious long-term effects on our health. Every time we decide to walk in the park, go for a swim or a run, or just choose the life option that makes us truly happy, we are doing our hearts good. Left neglected for too long, we run the risk not only physically of developing life-threatening diseases—particularly of arteries, the

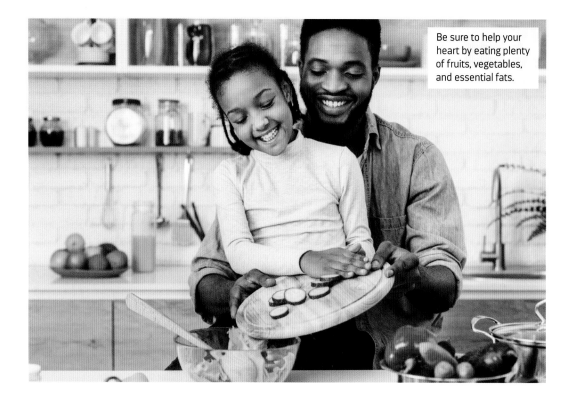

Be sure to help your heart by eating plenty of fruits, vegetables, and essential fats.

blood vessels that supply all the body's cells with nutrients and oxygen—but also depression and anxiety. Diet and coping mechanisms are the first line of defense.

Starting with diet, reduce your intake of saturated fat and eat plenty of fresh fruit and vegetables, which are high in antioxidants, as well as magnesium, calcium, and potassium, which are all important heart nutrients. Foods that are rich in magnesium include tofu, beans, seeds, almonds, cashews, buckwheat, garlic, whole grains, green leafy vegetables, and potato skins—next time you have a baked potato, make sure you eat the whole thing.

Increase the amounts of essential fats, especially the omega-3 essential fats, found in oily fish such as salmon, mackerel, tuna, herring, linseeds, walnuts, pumpkin seeds, soya, and green leafy vegetables. Garlic can help lower the blood pressure by dilating the blood vessels, and can be added raw to natural low-fat yogurt.

Antioxidant nutrients, such as beta-carotene, selenium, Vitamin E, and Vitamin C are important in protecting against the development of heart disease. They help prevent something called free radical damage. Fats and cholesterol are particularly susceptible to free radical damage—damage caused by toxins like cigarette smoke. This "damaged" cholesterol is much more dangerous to the heart and circulation system.

In this section, I look at ways to treat heart problems such as hypertension and angina. The most effective herb for heart health is probably the hawthorn. Its berries and leaves can be used to make a range of natural remedies to improve heart health.

Add raw garlic to your diet to help regulate the circulatory system.

High Blood Pressure

Also known as hypertension, which can cause headaches, shortness of breath, and visual disturbances. Raw garlic is used as a tonic to the circulatory system—ensure that you get lots in your diet. Regular massage, especially around the shoulders, middle back, and chest area can be very beneficial. Use oils such as lavender and ylang ylang. Hawthorn berries can be used to treat heart problems. Gather in the autumn months when the hedgerows are full of the deep red fruit.

Hawthorn Berry Brandy

- Several handfuls hawthorn berries and leaves
- Brandy, as needed

1. Pack the hawthorn berries and leaves into a large glass jar.
2. Cover with brandy and leave in a cool dark place for two weeks.
3. Strain the liquid into dark bottles and take 2 tablespoons daily as a heart tonic.

Low Blood Pressure

Also known as hypotension, this is a rapid drop in blood pressure. Many people experience it when standing up quickly. It is important to stimulate the circulation to avoid dizziness and fainting. Regular aerobic exercise is a good idea for everyone, but especially those suffering from hypotension. If you feel faint when you stand up quickly, lower your chin to your chest until the feeling subsides. Warming herbs such as rosemary and ginger are useful and can be made into a tea. (See Warming Ginger Tea recipe on page 50.) Massage with warming oils, such as black pepper and rosemary to help stimulate and warm the body.

Anemia

This is usually caused by an iron deficiency either through surgery, trauma, or childbirth. Nettle tea is an excellent tonic for those suffering from anemia.

Nettle Tea

- Handful young nettle tops
- Boiling water, as needed

1. Put on a pair of gloves and collect a handful of young nettle tops.
2. Place in a cup, pour over boiling water.
3. Place a plate over the top and leave to infuse for ten minutes.
4. Strain and drink while still warm.

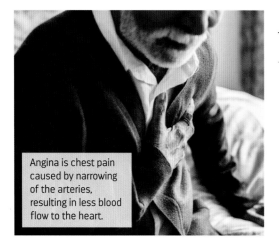

Angina is chest pain caused by narrowing of the arteries, resulting in less blood flow to the heart.

Angina

Angina is chest pain caused by the narrowing of the arteries. Pain occurs after exertion or a heavy meal. Motherwort is a wild plant that helps to calm the heart. It can be taken as a tea (see page 140). Hawthorn is another good treatment for angina. Make an infusion of the berries and take as a tonic.

Hawthorn Infusion

- Handful hawthorn berries and leaves
- Boiling water, as needed

1. Place the hawthorn berries and leaves into a cup. Pour boiling water to cover.
2. Leave to infuse for ten minutes.
3. Strain and drink. Enjoy three cups a day as a heart tonic.

Hemorrhoids

The primary cause of hemorrhoids is chronic constipation, straining, and the pressure this causes on the surrounding veins. Hemorrhoids are common during pregnancy and in conditions affecting the liver and upper bowel. Pain at passing stools, slight bleeding in the case of internal trouble, and feeling of soreness and irritation after passing a stool are the usual symptoms.

Cut a slim piece of potato and insert it into the anus to ease discomfort. Use witch hazel to make a compress and sit on it to reduce inflammation and swelling. Add rosemary essential oil to a warm bath as a soothing treatment before bed. Hemorrhoids can also be treated using the appropriately named pilewort. This plant is also known as lesser celandine (not to be confused with greater celandine) and can be found in wooded areas in the spring.

Pilewort Compress

- 1 ounce (25 g) pilewort root
- 18 fluid ounces (500 ml) water

1. Place the pilewort root into a saucepan and pour over the water.

2. Simmer gently for ten minutes.

3. Allow to cool and then strain.

4. Soak a cloth in the liquid and apply to the affected area. You can leave it on for half an hour, re-soaking the cloth as needed.

There are several natural remedies to help ease aching varicose veins.

Varicose Veins

Swollen veins, often occurring in the legs or in the rectum (hemorrhoids) are called varicose veins. Drink beetroot juice daily as it is strengthening to the system. Massage legs affected by varicose veins with a rosemary blend. A witch hazel compress can also ease aching varicose veins.

Massage Oil for Varicose Veins

Soothe the affected area with this nourishing oil blend.

- 1 cup organic sweet almond oil
- 3 drops rosemary essential oil

Using long strokes, massage into the affected area daily.

Witch Hazel Compress

- 1 ounce (25 g) cut witch hazel bark
- 18 fluid ounces (500 ml) water

1. Place the witch hazel bark into a saucepan and pour over the water.
2. Simmer gently for ten minutes.
3. Allow to cool and then strain.
4. Soak a cloth in the liquid and apply to the affected area. You can leave it on for half an hour, re-soaking the cloth as needed.

Plant Profile: Hawthorn

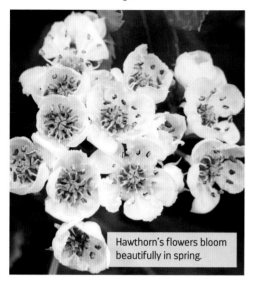

Hawthorn's flowers bloom beautifully in spring.

Hawthorn (*crataegus*) is synonymous with mid spring and is steeped in magic and mystery. With its beautiful flowers and sharp thorns, the hawthorn is a paradox of a plant. It has long been revered for its magical properties and has been loved and respected throughout history. It is found throughout Britain, Europe, western Asia, and North Africa and grows to between 5½–16½ yards (5–15 meters) tall. It is popular as a hedge plant and many animals and birds make their homes in its dense thorny twigs. The fruit are sometimes known as "haws", which is where the hawthorn gets its name. The thorns are usually ½–1 inch (1–3 cm) long, so you know when you've been pricked by one!

Hawthorns have been known to live for 400 years and clumps of twisted old trees can be found in towns, reminders of where old hedgerows were situated. The light, hard wood from the Hawthorn provides the hottest fire known.

Hawthorn is the sixth tree of the Celtic Tree Ogham. It represents love, fertility, the heart, protection, the release of blocked energy, and preparation for spiritual growth. For this reason, hawthorn has an affinity with the Celtic festival Beltane—the Hawthorn's Spring blossom was used to decorate and celebrate this fertile time of year. Before the church discredited spring customs, Hawthorn played a valuable part in May Day celebrations, when the union of the May Queen and the Green Man blessed the fertility of the Earth.

However, the folk customs lived on, and marriages continued to take place at this special, abundant time of year. Newly married couples would find garlands of mayflowers decorating their beds, representing fertility and lasting love. The maypole was traditionally a living Hawthorn tree, brought into the village and danced around to bring life, love, and fertility to a community.

Hawthorn trees are steeped in folklore and mythology.

Hawthorn branches were twisted into globes, or even made into crowns for protection.

A sprig of Hawthorn is said to promote happiness in the troubled, depressed, or sad.

Legend has it that young women bathed in the dew of Hawthorn as a beauty aid. Hawthorn has long been associated with the fairy realm, and there is much lore and legend surrounding it. A tea made of the leaves and blossoms is said to aid anxiety, appetite loss, and poor circulation, and this special plant has strong links with spirituality. Solitary hawthorns often marked old sacred groves or meeting places, wells, springs, underground water, and fairy places. Where groups of hawthorn trees grew in threes, they would be treated with great respect. Enchantment was said to be the result of lingering under these trees. It has long been considered bad luck to uproot or disturb a hawthorn tree and cuttings were only made on May 1st, or Beltane.

Hawthorn is also recognized as a protective plant and charms were made by twisting the branches into globes, which were hung in houses and in babies' cradles. In Ireland, people would tie ribbons and rags ("clouties") to hawthorn trees situated near sacred wells, as gifts to the fairies and tree spirits. These gifts were said to attract love and healing to the giver and symbolize a wish made. A pink ribbon was used to wish for love, a blue ribbon to wish for protection, a green ribbon to wish for wealth and a purple or indigo ribbon to wish for greater knowledge. Love and respect for this plant did not die out with the arrival of the Christians—Jesus' crown of thorns was said to be a wreath of Hawthorn and the Burning Bush seen by Moses a hawthorn bush.

Hawthorn also has culinary and herbal uses. The berries have been used as a cardiac tonic for centuries and the leaves as a substitute for oriental green tea. A tea made of the leaves and blossoms is said to aid anxiety, appetite loss, and poor circulation. Dried hawthorn berries are used as a digestive aid in naturopathic and traditional Chinese medicine. Hawthorn is also used as an aid to lower blood pressure and treat some heart-related diseases. The haws are often used to make jams, which are considered a delicacy.

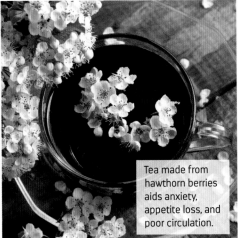

Tea made from hawthorn berries aids anxiety, appetite loss, and poor circulation.

BONES, MUSCLES, AND JOINTS

OUR BONES, MUSCLES, AND JOINTS CAN BE SUBJECT TO INJURY, SO IT IS important that we look after them and take appropriate care when damage does occur. At the first sign of injury, bruising, accident, or pain, take homeopathic remedy Arnica 30. This will help your body cope with the shock and reduce swelling and ease bruising.

Pain can be more acute when our bodies go into a state of shock and we forget to drink water. Dehydration makes pain worse as muscles create acidic waste when in pain. Drinking two glasses of water as soon as the pain comes on will help stop this painful waste building up and give almost immediate relief. Cold packs are also great for reducing inflammation, soothing away pain, and aiding recovery—use a pack of frozen peas and press to the affected area.

The diet is also important in maintaining good muscle and joint health; essential fatty acids are great for increasing muscle flexibility and repairing muscle tissue. Make sure your diet is rich in the right kinds of fatty acids such as oily fish, hemp, and flaxseed oil.

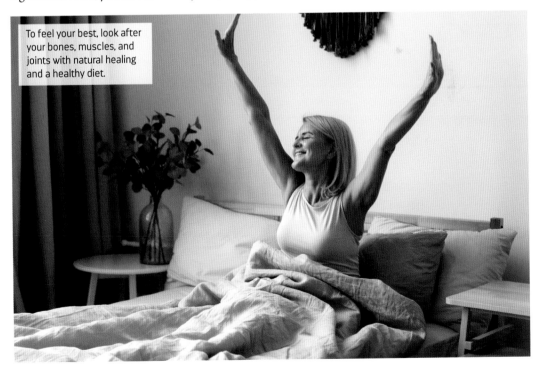

To feel your best, look after your bones, muscles, and joints with natural healing and a healthy diet.

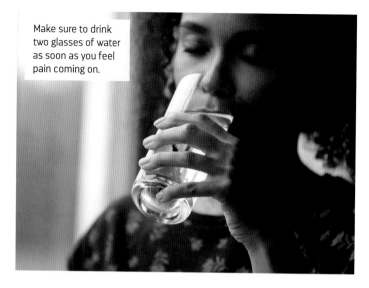

Make sure to drink two glasses of water as soon as you feel pain coming on.

There are many plants that can be used in the treatment of aches and pains—find out how to make seaweed liniment to treat arthritis and brew up your own cider vinegar which can be used to treat a host of conditions from sprains to skin disorders, digestive upset to urinary infections.

Osteoporosis

Osteoporosis is when the bones lose their density with age and become more porous. It can mean that fractures and breakages in the bones are more likely. Eat plenty of calcium, and rich wild greens such as nettles and dandelion. The leaves of both can be made into a tea or added to soups and stews. To make a tea, simply take a handful of fresh leaves of either plant, place in a cup, add boiling water, and leave to steep for ten minutes. Drink three cups a day if needed.

Comfrey is an excellent tonic for bone health—the folk name for comfrey is in fact "knitbone". The leaves can be harvested in the spring and summer and dried to make a medicinal tea.

Comfrey Tea

Once you pick your comfrey leaves, tie the stems together and hang in a dry spot until the leaves have dried. Then cut off the stems and place the leaves in a jar.

- 1 tablespoon dried comfrey leaves
- Boiling water, as needed

1. Take 1 tablespoon of the dried herb and place in a cup.
2. Add boiling water, cover, and allow to steep for five minutes.
3. Drink up to three cups a day.

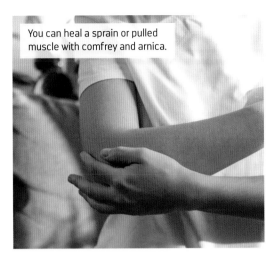

You can heal a sprain or pulled muscle with comfrey and arnica.

Sprains and Pulled Muscles

These occur generally after over-stretching often caused during sports. Comfrey and arnica are effective at treating areas of damaged tissue such as a sprain. Apply an ointment or gently massage comfrey oil (see page 109) into the sore area. It is not a good idea to use either of these herbs in cases of broken skin. Make up a potent massage oil using eucalyptus, lavender, and rosemary essential oils. Apple cider vinegar can be used as a cold compress on the affected limb to reduce swelling and relieve pain. You can make your own apple cider vinegar, which is also useful in the treatment of skin disorders, digestive troubles, urinary infections, and illnesses of the respiratory system. (Recipe for Apple Cider Vinegar on page 109.)

Massage Oil for Sprains

Make up this massage blend to treat sprains—can also be added to a warm bath for relief.

- 1½ fluid ounces (30 ml) carrier oil, such as organic sweet almond oil
- 2 drops each eucalyptus, lavender, and rosemary essential oils

Mix all ingredients together and apply twice daily to the sprained muscle.

Squeeze aloe vera juice into a glass of warm water and drink to help the bones heal after a fracture.

Fractures

Often the result of injury, a fracture is a break or crack in the bone. The homeopathic remedy Arnica and a few drops of rescue remedy should be taken at the time of injury. After the injury, take aloe vera internally to help the body heal. Squeeze the juice from one leaf into a glass of warm water or fruit juice, blend, and drink. Take comfrey tea regularly after injury to help the bones to heal (see recipe on opposite page). The fractured joint can also be massaged with comfrey oil (see recipe on page 109), as long as the skin is not broken.

Rheumatism

Rheumatism is an umbrella term that covers aches, pains, and stiffness in the bones and muscles. Horseradish is said to prevent attacks of rheumatism—pick a leaf and chew it slowly. Seaweed can be harvested and made into a liniment to treat rheumatism. Rose petals can be added to running water to make a soothing bath for rheumatic pain—simply add a handful and step in. A wonderful warming oil can be made from cayenne, which can be used to treat aches, pains, and stiffness.

Cayenne Oil

- 1 tablespoon cayenne pepper
- 2 tablespoons crushed mustard seed
- 2 teaspoons grated ginger root
- 8 fluid ounces (250 ml) sunflower oil

1. Mix all the ingredients in a glass jar.

2. Leave to infuse for one week.

3. Massage into the affected area to treat muscle spasms and stiff joints.

Seaweed Liniment

- 1 ounce (25 g) bladderwrack (from the beach)
- 18 fluid ounces (500 ml) water
- Comfrey oil (see recipe on page 109)

1. Place the bladderwrack in a saucepan and pour the water over.

2. Simmer gently for thirty minutes.

3. Strain and measure the liquid.

4. Add an equal volume of comfrey oil.

5. Shake well before use. Rub into infected areas, morning and night.

Bladderwrack, a medicinal sea algae.

To prevent backaches, plan a fun dance class that will encourage you to exercise.

Backache

We often take our spines completely for granted until something happens to arrest their mobility. Whether caused by a fall, a bump, an awkward twist, or just sheer buildup of stress, pain in the back leaves us crying out for relief and often unable to move. Most of us experience backache at some point in our lives. With an increasingly sedentary lifestyle consisting of a great deal of time spent sitting in the same position in office chairs staring at a computer screen it is hardly surprising that back pain is on the rise. Fortunately, there are many ways to promote health of the spine and prevent back pain in the first place.

Regular exercise is very beneficial for the health of the spine. Yoga or Pilates are particularly helpful in stretching and releasing any areas of tension before they build up and become painful. Try to incorporate a daily stretching session and at least thirty minutes of walking into your day. Ideally you would combine this with a session of aerobic exercise such as swimming, cycling, or running. It is a good idea to aim to get your heart pumping at least once a day. Plan exercise sessions that are fun and that you can do with friends, such as a group cycle ride/walk or a dance class, which will help you to stick to them.

There are also plenty of natural remedies that can be used to treat discomfort in the back. Make up a massage oil using a base of 7 fluid ounces (200 ml) organic sweet almond oil with two drops each of rosemary, lavender, and eucalyptus. This can be massaged into the affected area or added to a warm bath to soothe and ease pain. Chew on a small horseradish leaf to help relieve the pain. Apply a mustard poultice to the affected area to ease pain and help release blockages in the back.

Mustard Poultice

- ½ teaspoon mustard seeds
- 1 tablespoon plain flour
- Warm water, as needed

1. Place the mustard seed and flour in a bowl. Add enough warm water to form a paste.

2. Spread the mixture over one half of a flannel and fold the flannel over so that it is covered.

3. Wear a cotton t-shirt or cover your back with a cotton sheet and place the wrapped poultice over the affected area.

4. Leave the poultice on for an hour, checking regularly that the skin hasn't become red or sore (some people have very sensitive skin and find mustard too strong). If the skin is red and uncomfortable, remove the poultice and wash with cool water.

Arthritis

Arthritis is inflammation of the tissues surrounding the joints. Pain, swelling, and redness usually result. Nettles are a traditional remedy for arthritis and can be use in cookery or made into a tea. A glass of water with 1 teaspoon of honey and 1 tablespoon of vinegar is a soothing remedy to ease the pain. Also add apple cider vinegar to a warm bath to promote healing—you can make your own by fermenting apple juice (see opposite page). Make a homemade seaweed liniment to treat arthritis or rheumatism.

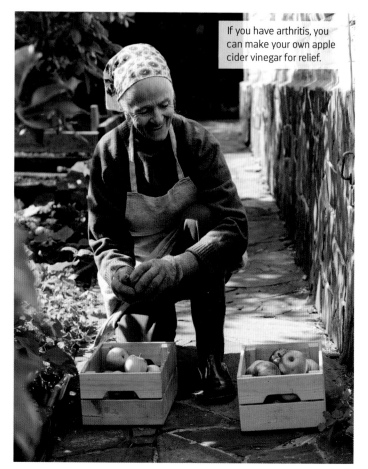

If you have arthritis, you can make your own apple cider vinegar for relief.

Comfrey Oil

- 1 handful dried comfrey leaves
- Sweet almond oil or apricot oil, as needed

1. Place the comfrey leaves in a glass jar with a lid and cover completely with the oil.

2. Seal and leave to infuse for four to eight weeks, shaking daily.

3. When the oil has turned a deeper color, strain through a piece of muslin and pour into a dark glass bottle.

4. Store in the refrigerator and use on its own to treat muscle pain, sprains, and broken bones or add to the Seaweed Liniment on page 106.

Apple Cider Vinegar

Use fully ripe, unbruised apples and avoid metal utensils or containers when making or storing the vinegar as the acid will react to the metal. The number of apples needed will depend on their size, so you may need to adjust the quantities given here depending on how much juice your apples yield. This recipe is for 3½ pints (2 liters) of apple cider vinegar.

1. Quarter, then crush the apples and strain the pulp through a piece of muslin cloth, reserving the juice.

2. To make the starter, remove 8 fluid ounces (250 ml) of the juice and add a square of winemaker's yeast (refer to the packaging for exact quantity needed).

3. Mix thoroughly and stir into the rest of the juice.

4. Pour the mixture into a large glass bowl or lidless container. Cover with a piece of muslin cloth and store out of direct sunlight for three to four weeks at a temperature between 61°F and 35.5°F (16°C and 26°C). Stir the mixture daily.

5. After three weeks, taste the vinegar. If it is not strong enough, wait another week. When you are happy with the flavor, strain the vinegar and pasteurize it by heating to 140°F (60°C) in a saucepan.

6. Pour into clean bottles with airtight lids. Place the sealed bottles in a pan filled with hot water. Allow the water to cool and then store.

Plant Profile: Comfrey

Comfrey is a wonderful plant native to Europe that has a myriad of uses, not least in your garden. In fact, it has been said that comfrey has more uses than any other herb. The roots can grow up to ten feet deep and draw the nutrients from deep in the soil up to ground level, into the subsoil to feed other neighboring plants and to enrich the soil. Nutrients, minerals, and moisture are transported in this way by a herb that is often grown as green manure (a plant that enriches the soil during growth and is then dug into the earth to give further nutrients at the end of the growing period) because of its beneficial effect on the soil and its usefulness as cattle feed. The plant can be recognized by its large bristly leaves and purple flower clusters in the summertime.

Comfrey has many healing properties and makes a great addition to your garden.

Some consider comfrey a weed, but organic gardeners are well aware of its value. To make a nutrient-rich spray for the garden, loosely fill a bucket with cut leaves and top up with water.

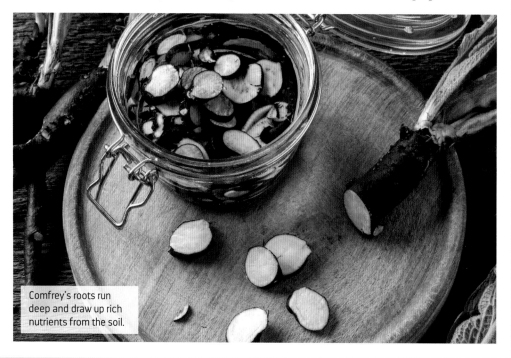

Comfrey's roots run deep and draw up rich nutrients from the soil.

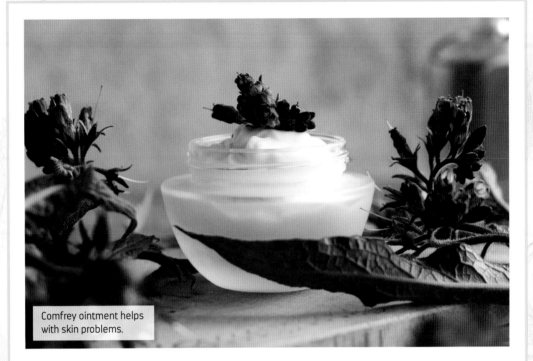

Comfrey ointment helps with skin problems.

Press down and leave for a few weeks. It will look and smell horrible, but the resulting deep-brown liquid can be diluted and decanted into a spray bottle to use on tomatoes, onions, and beans. Another use for comfrey in the garden is as a slug repellent. You can place cut leaves in a heap encouraging slugs to eat these instead of your new seedlings. The leaves can also be placed around the base of a plant and hopefully the slugs will feast on these before attacking your vegetables.

Laurence Hills, the founder of the Henry Doubleday Research Association (now known as Garden Organic), devoted all his early work to research and experimentation with comfrey. He suggested that every organic garden should continuously have a patch of comfrey growing. Hills recommends mixing the leaves into the compost heap as an activator.

Although it has a bitter taste, comfrey is often enjoyed by humans as well as slugs and can be served in salads or steamed lightly and cooked as a green vegetable. It also makes a good base for detoxifying green drinks containing other superfoods such as spirulina. It is a rich source of Vitamin B12 and has more protein in its leaf structure than any other plant. It is an excellent detoxicant and has a cleansing effect on the liver and lung tissues. Even the root can be used to make a coffee substitute much like dandelion or chicory.

Traditional folk names for comfrey include "knitbone" or "boneset" due to its healing properties and use for treating broken bones by early herbalists. Today the plant is used to make an ointment that is effective in treating skin problems and bruising. Lastly the leaves can also be used to make a beautiful yellow dye. So this really is one plant that you can put to use in every area of your house and garden.

Eyes and Ears

LOOKING AFTER YOUR PRIME SENSE
organs is vital. There are several natural
remedies that can be used to treat common
problems with the eyes, such as conjunctivitis
and eyestrain. The most widely recognized herb
for addressing eye problems is eyebright, or
Euphrasia officinalis. Found throughout Europe,
this herb has been used since the Middle Ages
to treat bloodshot and irritated eyes. The flowers,
which have spots and stripes, are thought to
resemble bloodshot eyes, and followers of the
Doctrine of Signatures believe that plants exhibit
signs of the symptoms they can be used to treat.

Eyebright is an herb
that most commonly
addresses eye problems.

To reduce eyestrain,
take a walk and look out
towards the horizon.

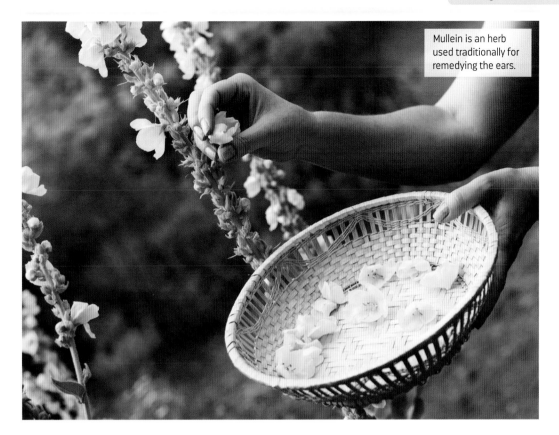

Mullein is an herb used traditionally for remedying the ears.

On the following pages you can learn how to make an eye-brightening infusion which can be used to treat conjunctivitis, styes, and eyestrain. Modern lifestyles often involve spending a great deal of time in front of a computer screen or focusing on objects close to us, causing our eyes to suffer from tiredness. Make sure that they get adequate rest and that you spend time every day looking into the distance.

Our ancestors would have spent much of their time watching the horizon and looking at things far away. It is thought that increasing levels of myopia (or short-sightedness) are in part caused by our tendency to focus on the small things in front of us. It is a good idea to take a fifteen-minute walk every day and really focus on the horizon while you are walking. You can also try an eye yoga exercise to relieve tired eyes. Rub your palms together vigorously to create heat, then place your palms over your eyes for several minutes and breathe deeply.

The ears are prone to infection when there is a buildup of mucus in the system, and this can be treated using garlic and raw onion. Another traditional remedy for the ears is mullein, a beautiful tall plant with a spike of big blousy flowers. In this chapter, you'll find out how to make your own mullein oil, which can be used to treat infection and buildup of wax.

Conjunctivitis

Conjunctivitis is inflammation of the mucus membrane that lines the eyelids and covers the outer layer of the eyeball. It can be a reaction to allergens in the atmosphere, such as pollens, or cosmetics. Dilute a tablespoon of honey in a cup of warm water to make an eye bath that will cleanse the area, treat an infection, and promote healing. Make an eye wash using a cup of tepid chamomile tea. A cotton pad can be used to cleanse the eye. Make sure that you use a new pad for each eye to reduce the risk of spreading the infection. Lavender, chamomile, or rose essential oil can be added to warm water to make a soothing eye bath that will draw out the infection.

Soothing Eye Bath

Cleanse the infected eye with a cotton pad soaked in this soothing wash.

- 1 cup warm water
- 1 drop lavender oil, chamomile, or rose essential oil

1. Mix ingredients together and soak a cotton wool pad in the warm liquid.
2. Apply to infected eye. Use at least twice daily.

Eyebright Infusion

Use infusion of eyebright to help restore health to itchy, infected eyes.

- 4 mg dried eyebright
- 1 cup boiled water

1. Soak the eyebright in the boiled water for ten minutes.
2. Strain and cool.
3. Using a clean flannel, bathe the eyes with this infusion twice a day.

Eyestrain

After staring at a screen for several hours your eyes can become tired and feel irritated. Add 2 drops of rose essential oil to 2 tablespoons carrier oil, such as organic olive oil, and massage into the temples to relieve tension. You can also make an infusion using rose petals. Place slices of cucumber over the eyes to calm and soothe the eye area. Make a compress from an infusion of chickweed to ease tired, sore eyes.

Rose Petal Infusion

To combat sore, tired eyes, make this wonderfully relaxing rose petal tea.

- 1 cup water, just off the boil
- 1 handful rose petals, preferably organic or wild

1. Place the rose petals in the hot water.
2. Cover and leave to infuse for ten minutes.
3. Strain the resulting warm liquid and use it to bathe your eyes.

Chickweed Infusion

- 1 handful chickweed leaves
- 2 cups boiling water

1. Place the chickweed leaves into a teapot. Add the boiling water.
2. Leave for ten minutes, then strain.
3. Soak a cloth in the liquid, fold into a rectangle, and rest over the eyes for ten minutes.

Styes

A stye is a small yellow blister at the base of the eyelash that occurs when the immune system is compromised. See remedies for Conjunctivitis on page 114 to soothe any irritation. A calendula tincture can also be applied topically to reduce swelling and taken internally to support the immune system. Dilute 1 tablespoon of tincture to a cup of warm water and drink up to three times a day.

Calendula Tincture

- 1 large handful fresh calendula flowers
- 7 fluid ounces (200 ml) alcohol, such as organic vodka
- 3½ fluid ounces (100 ml) water

1. Place the flowers in a large glass jar.
2. Cover with the alcohol and water.
3. Replace the lid and leave for two weeks, shaking occasionally.
4. Strain through a sieve with a muslin cloth placed inside.
5. Pour the liquid into a clean dark glass bottle and store for up to a year.

Ear Wax Buildup

Hard wax sometimes accumulates in the ear and an excess can obstruct the canal and affect hearing. This condition can be made worse by swimming as the wax absorbs water. Warm some mullein oil and place a few drops into the ear canal.

Placing raw garlic or onion inside your ear will help draw out an ear infection.

Middle Ear Infection

An ear infection is sometimes a side effect of a sore throat or chesty cold, often accompanied by fever. Use garlic extensively in the diet to help the body rid itself of infection. You can also place a piece of cut, peeled garlic wrapped in gauze directly into the ear to treat the infection. Naturopaths often recommend a slice of raw onion placed around the ear to draw out infection. Leave it in place for as long as possible and replace when it has dried out.

Yarrow Infusion

- ½ cup boiling water
- 1 handful yarrow plant—leaves and flowers

1. Place yarrow in a heatproof container. Pour over boiling water.
2. Leave to steep for ten minutes, covered.
3. Pour warm infusion into the affected ear. Can also use a pipette to apply the infusion, to avoid getting wet!

Massage lavender oil into the neck and throat area. Mullein is the herbal remedy for ears, and you can make an effective oil from this plant. Drop a pipette full into your ear canal and keep your head on one side to absorb.

Mullein Oil

- 1 mullein plant
- Organic sunflower oil, as needed

1. Break the flowering spike of the mullein plant into smaller pieces.
2. Place in a pestle and add a small amount of organic sunflower oil.
3. Crush with the mortar to start releasing the beneficial parts of the plant.
4. Place in a large glass jar.
5. Cover with more oil so that the plant is well covered, then put the lid on and shake well.
6. Leave outside in direct sunlight for twenty-one days.

Plant Profile: Fennel

Fennel (*Foeniculum vulgare*) is a perennial and umbelliferous plant, meaning that it has umbrella-like bursts of flowers on tall, upright stalks. The common garden fennel has soft, feathery foliage which smells of aniseed when crushed, and it looks very similar to the dill plant. The species Florence fennel possesses the swollen, bulb-like stem base, which is the familiar vegetable most often using in cooking. The thin, ovoid, grooved seeds are used extensively for their sweet, aniseed flavor. Fennel is indigenous to Europe but cultivated in India, China, and Egypt.

Fennel's rich and interesting history is chronicled in herbal folklore. The Ancient Greeks valued fennel highly—one of their most famous cities, Marathon (which translates as "fennel") was so named because of the abundance of the aromatic herb growing there. The Romans cultivated the plant for its edible shoots and seeds and recorded its use to sharpen the sight of snakes. Mediaeval English herbalists prized it for many reasons, including its professed power to ward away evil. Fennel features in the pagan Anglo-Saxon Nine Herbs Charm, recorded in the tenth century. This fascinating charm was intended for the treatment of poison and infection through the preparation of nine herbs.

Fennel crops up in the culinary traditions of many different cultures. The bulb of Florence fennel is popular in Mediterranean countries where it features in salads, pastas, and risottos, along with the tasty fronds. The Chinese use fennel in their five-spice powder and the seeds are an integral part of the flavors of many Indian and Middle Eastern dishes.

As a medicinal herb, fennel is perhaps best known for its digestive carminative properties. Try bruising a teaspoon of fennel seeds and adding boiling water to make a soothing and

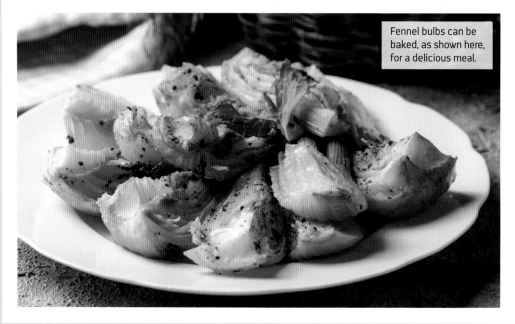

Fennel bulbs can be baked, as shown here, for a delicious meal.

Fennel can aid eyesight, bloating, breastfeeding, and more.

You can use fennel seeds or essential oils for natural healing.

antispasmodic tea. This creates an excellent tonic to ease bloating, indigestion, and flatulence. Fennel was traditionally mixed with sodium bicarbonate and syrup to make gripe water, given to babies to ease painful colic. As far back as Ancient Greece, fennel was used as a slimming aid as it can suppress the appetite.

Fennel has a long history of use for the treatment of eye problems, and on the Indian subcontinent fennel seeds are often eaten raw to improve eyesight. A fennel compress can help with conjunctivitis and blepharitis. As a folk remedy, fennel has been used for jaundice, hepatitis, and other liver disorders as it is said to restore damaged liver cells. To help cleanse the liver, drink a tea made with one teaspoon of bruised fennel seed or two teaspoons of finely chopped fresh leaves to a cup of boiling water.

Breastfeeding mothers find the gifts of fennel to be manifold. It works as a galactagogue, improving milk flow in a gentle and safe way. A cooling compress made with bruised fennel seeds can be used for engorged and painful breasts. The plant contains phytoestrogens—plant compounds that exert a balancing effect on female hormone levels. This makes it an ideal companion throughout life and many women find it very helpful for hormonal upsets ranging from PMS to menopause. There is reported use of fennel to enlarge the breasts dating back to Roman times when it was also used to increase the libido. Although there are no guarantees, drinking fennel tea is a far more holistic option than surgery!

WOMEN'S HEALTH

*

As women, we are blessed with amazing bodies that follow the cycles of the moon in our menstruation, can carry, nurture, and give birth to babies, and then provide the perfect nutrients in the form of breast milk for our children. In our medicalized society it is possible to forget the power and strength of our bodies.

Periods, pregnancy, birth, and menopause all show the strength of a woman's body.

Doing yoga while pregnant can help you become more in tune with your body's needs.

We may take medication to control the menstrual period or even eliminate it altogether. When pregnant, we often forget to trust our instincts and listen to what our bodies need and may not take time to marvel at the miracle happening inside us, and when labor kicks in most doctors and midwives advise the mother to go to the hospital to be helped to give birth.

This is the norm in our society, but many women are starting to question it and look outside the mainstream for alternatives. Of course, medical help is an essential part of giving birth and modern medicine can aid the various hormonal transitions women go through, but nature also offers us a wealth of ways to help with these natural processes. When we can embrace our monthly bleeding and the possible emotions that come up with it, rather than trying to control it, we may find that the strain and pain is lessened.

When we can trust our innate ability to birth and nurture our young, working with our bodies as nature intended, we can rediscover the amazing power we have to create new life. This section is all about women's bodies and ways to treat our life processes such as periods, pregnancy, birth, and menopause naturally.

Consult a doctor if you find a lump on your breast or any other part of your body.

MENSTRUAL CYCLE

SINCE ANCIENT TIMES IT HAS BEEN BELIEVED THAT MENSTRUAL CYCLES ARE connected to the moon, causing women to bleed at the dark (or new) moon and ovulate when the moon is full. Many women have problems with their menstrual cycle, but there are a host of natural remedies that can be used to create a balance.

Dysmenorrhea is the name given to painful periods, while menorrhagia means heavy bleeding, and the absence of periods is known as amenorrhea. Many women suffer with period pain every month, and this could, in part, be due to our culture. Periods are often seen as something shameful, to be hidden and to be suffered. It is not often that we allow ourselves to rest and take time out during our monthly bleed, although this is practiced by some tribal cultures around the world even today. While the demands of modern life may not allow us complete rest, even in today's fast-paced society we can incorporate a time of relaxation into our everyday lives.

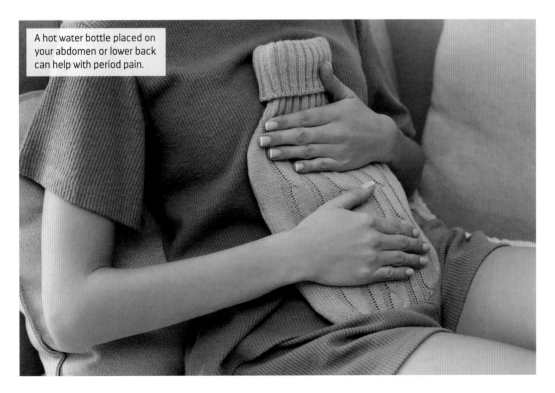

A hot water bottle placed on your abdomen or lower back can help with period pain.

Promise yourself an afternoon in bed, a lie-in, or an early night at the start of your period. Indulge your taste buds—what would you like to eat now? Treat yourself and let go of guilt. Make your own comfort your maximum priority—are you warm enough? Do you need an extra blanket? More pillows? Would you like a hot water bottle placed on your abdomen or lower back? It may be helpful to mark when your cycle begins on a calendar or in a diary and note how you feel each day, remembering that self-care during this time of the month is vital. Once you get into the flow of this you may start to notice an easing of your usual symptoms. Peppermint tea can help to ease bloating and pain during menstruation. Make a massage oil with a few drops each of clary sage and fennel essential oils to regulate the hormones.

Moontime Massage Oil

Mix up this calming blend before your period starts to help balance your hormones.

- 1½ fluid ounces (30 ml) carrier oil, such as organic sweet almond oil
- 2 drops clary sage essential oil
- 2 drops fennel essential oil

1. Mix ingredients together in an amber bottle.

2. Massage into lower back and abdomen with long sweeping strokes to ease discomfort.

3. Use as often as needed in the lead up to, and during your period.

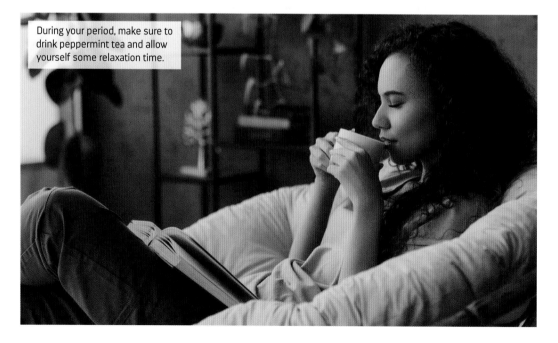

During your period, make sure to drink peppermint tea and allow yourself some relaxation time.

FERTILITY

FERTILITY HAS BECOME A SUBJECT OF huge anxiety for many women throughout the Western world. But the impulse to turn to drugs and invasive medical procedures is in many cases unnecessary. Alternative therapies have been found to be extremely effective in correcting and restoring full reproductive function.

Firstly, diet is extremely important in reproductive health. Vitamin C, selenium, and zinc are particularly important. Zinc is critical for maintaining optimum levels of semen, and essential for the functioning of male and female reproductive organs—it is also one of the minerals most depleted by sustained stress levels and toxic lifestyles. Vitamin C is important in sperm production, as it improves mobility.

Fertility issues affect many people. With the help of alternative therapies, full reproductive function can be restored.

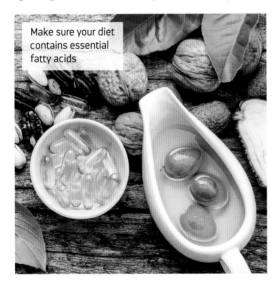

Make sure your diet contains essential fatty acids

Selenium deficiencies have been linked to reduced sperm counts and sterility in men and infertility in women. This mineral can be found in Brazil nuts so ensure that these tasty nuts are a regular part of your diet.

Cutting down on toxins will boost vitality, libido, and fertility. Alcohol and tobacco are known to reduce sperm count and can prevent implantation of the fertilized egg in women. Fried, fatty foods, sugar, and caffeine should be limited or eliminated if possible. A diet high in essential fatty acids (found in flax, hemp, oily fish, and pumpkin seeds) has been shown to be beneficial.

PREGNANCY

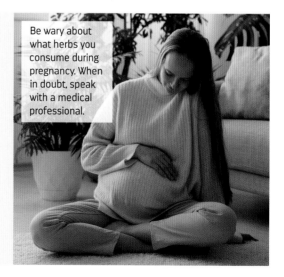

Most alternative medicines have no negative side effects in pregnancy. However, when in doubt, speak to a medical professional.

PREGNANCY IS THE START OF THE parenting journey. It is an incredible period of creativity and change during which it is important to nurture both body and mind. A woman's body is often optimally healthy during pregnancy and this state of health can be encouraged through a good diet and holistic therapies. There is a natural tendency for self-healing when minor illnesses or imbalances occur. Natural therapies can work with the body to enhance and strengthen this ability. If used appropriately, most alternative medicines have no dangerous or unpleasant side effects and are safe for use in pregnancy, however some herbs and herbal remedies are best avoided during pregnancy. If you are in any doubt, always check with a trained herbalist or doctor.

CAUTION:
Herbs to Avoid in Pregnancy

Many herbs and herbal remedies can be used safely throughout pregnancy to offer natural relief from the various discomforts and ailments that may occur. However, some herbs should be avoided. It is a good idea to consult an herbalist or get hold of a book that specifically deals with using herbs during pregnancy to help you identify those plants that are not safe for use at this special time.

Be wary about what herbs you consume during pregnancy. When in doubt, speak with a medical professional.

Pregnancy Anemia

Low iron levels in the blood can cause feelings of weakness, dizziness, and fainting. Take red raspberry leaf tea (page 128), which contains iron that is easily assimilated into the system. This is best avoided until the final trimester however, as raspberry can cause the uterus to contract. When eating foods containing iron, such as watercress, pumpkin seeds, and oats, remember that Vitamin C, found in many fruits and green vegetables, is needed by the body to break down the iron.

Yoga can help with posture in pregnancy. However, not all poses are suitable for pregnant women.

Pregnancy Backache

Backache can be caused by changes in your posture needed to accommodate the baby's weight. Try to stand straight and tall and wear comfortable shoes. Yoga and Pilates can be very beneficial in helping to encourage a better posture. Poses such as Cat stretch and Two Foot Support can help you to really become aware of the spine and its correct alignment, but be aware that not all poses are suitable for pregnant women.

Soothing Massage Oil

This is a good massage oil for backache during pregnancy and a useful tool for easing aches and pains.

- 2 drops rose essential oil
- 2 drops geranium essential oil
- 2 drops lavender essential oil
- 2 drops Roman chamomile essential oil
- 1½ fluid ounces (30 ml) sweet almond oil

1. Drop the essential oils into a glass jar.

2. Add the sweet almond oil and shake to mix.

3. Use as a massage treatment or add a capful to warm running water for a soothing bath.

Pregnancy Constipation

Constipation is the difficulty in passing stools sometimes caused by over-the-counter iron supplements. Cut back on wheat products, eat more dried fruits, and take more fluids. As some prescription iron supplements can have a constipating effect, try an iron-rich tonic such as Floradix or make yourself some nettle tea, which is naturally rich in iron.

Bleeding Gums

Hormonal changes can lead to a softening of the gum tissue, which is more easily damaged during pregnancy. Increase your Vitamin C intake to help your body heal and to strengthen the gums. Red raspberry leaf tea is also good for treating bleeding gums, but limit the use of this herb to the third trimester.

Red Raspberry Leaf Tea

Only use this preparation in the third trimester of pregnancy.

- 1 cup boiling water
- 1 tablespoon dried raspberry leaves

1. Place raspberry leaves in a cup and add water just off the boil.
2. Cover and leave to steep for ten minutes.
3. Drink to strengthen your system. Can take up to three cups a day in the last trimester.

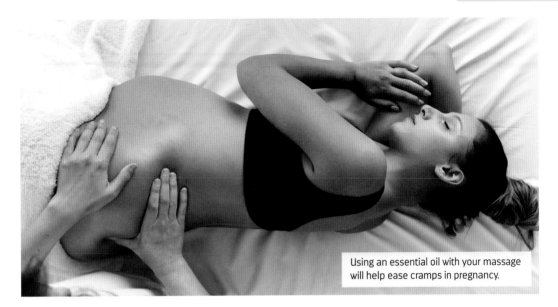

Using an essential oil with your massage will help ease cramps in pregnancy.

Cramps

During pregnancy, cramps occur mainly in the thighs, calves, and feet due to poor circulation or calcium deficiency. Eat plenty of garlic to improve circulation. A daily leg massage also helps prevent cramping at night. See page 127 for a soothing massage oil blend.

Pregnancy Indigestion

Indigestion is abdominal discomfort due to reduced capacity to digest food. Drink fennel tea and avoid rich, spicy, or fried foods. Yoga and Pilates can alleviate the pain caused by pressure on the diaphragm.

Fennel Tea

- 1 tablespoon dried fennel seeds
- Boiling water, as needed

1. Place the fennel seeds in a cup. Pour boiling water over to cover.
2. Place a plate on top to allow to infuse for ten minutes.
3. Drink after a meal to help the body digest more easily.

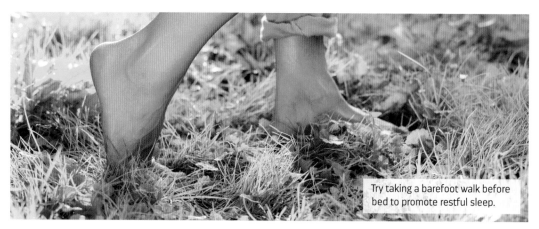

Try taking a barefoot walk before bed to promote restful sleep.

Pregnancy Insomnia

Discomfort near the end of pregnancy can make sleeping difficult. A teaspoon of honey and cider vinegar in warm water can help you get more restful sleep. Also try drinking celery juice. Daily exercise, preferably outdoors, is a real tonic for sleeplessness. Try a barefoot walk on the lawn before bed. It may sound silly, but it helps to discharge the electromagnetic charge that builds up during the day and helps to promote restful sleep. Take little naps during the day and avoid watching TV before you go to bed. In fact, switch off any electrical equipment at the wall. Also, make sure your bedroom is well ventilated.

Fluid Retention

The balance of salt and potassium in the cells causes hands, legs, and feet to swell. Massage can help to reduce water retention in the legs—try the massage oil blend on page 127.

Dizziness

Change position slowly so that your blood vessels have time to adjust and eat little and often.

Morning Sickness

Morning sickness is a feeling of nausea usually experienced in the first three months of pregnancy. Severe morning sickness may cause regular vomiting and is not necessarily confined to the morning. Ginger is very good for nausea. Try making a cup of ginger tea by steeping fresh ginger in hot water for ten minutes. Try homeopathic remedies—Ipecac for continued nausea not relieved by vomiting; Sepia if the nausea is made worse by the smell or thought of food; Nux Vomica for nausea that is worse in the morning; and Pulsatilla for nausea that comes on in the evening. When you must travel long distances when pregnant, wear a pair of travel bands on your wrists which work on acupressure points and are available from most good health food stores or chemists. Boost your levels of Vitamin B6, found in bananas, cereals, lentils, and fish.

Pelvic Pain

Pain in the pelvis caused by pressure on the pelvic nerves. Massage the thighs and pelvic area quite firmly to relieve muscle pain and tightness. See page 127 for a massage oil recipe.

Pregnancy Hemorrhoids

Hemorrhoids are caused by a body under stress through lack of nutrients. Apply an ice-cold witch hazel compress (see page 100) on gauze over the swelling.

Stretch Marks

These are fine red lines that eventually turn silver, caused by the skin stretching. Apply aloe vera gel directly from the succulent leaves onto your belly, breasts, and thighs to prevent stretch marks. Food containing zinc, such as sunflower and pumpkin seeds, can help to boost your skin's elasticity.

The gel from an aloe vera plant can prevent stretch marks.

Growing Bump Oil

- 3½ fluid ounces (100 ml) coconut oil
- 5 drops rose essential oil

1. Place the coconut oil and rose essential oil into a small glass bowl.

2. Warm slightly over a pan of boiling water.

3. Massage the warm, sweetly scented oil into your abdomen.

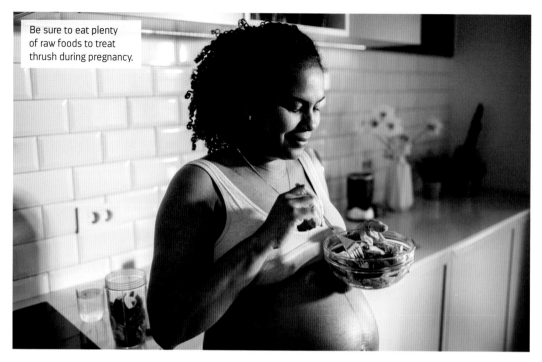

Be sure to eat plenty of raw foods to treat thrush during pregnancy.

Thrush

This vaginal infection is often caused by extra pressure on the immune system during pregnancy. Chamomile, fennel, and thyme can be used to treat thrush with their anti-fungal properties. Natural yogurt can also be applied. Eat plenty of raw foods, especially garlic. You can also massage olive oil liberally around the vulva and labia. Wear cotton underwear and avoid tight-fitting clothes. Cut out sugar and other sweeteners such as honey and molasses, as sugar distresses the immune system.

Chamomile, Fennel, and Thyme Infusion

These three herbs have anti-fungal properties.

- 1 large bowl water, just off the boil
- 1 tablespoon dried fennel
- 1 tablespoon dried thyme
- 1 tablespoon dried chamomile

1. Add the herbs to the large bowl and cover with water just off the boil. Cover and leave to steep for ten minutes.

2. Strain and soak an organic cotton or bamboo cloth in the tepid water. Make sure that it is warm. You don't want to cause any shock by applying a cold cloth.

3. Apply as a compress to the vulva.

Tiredness

Your body is creating a new human being—it is understandable that you will feel more tired than usual. Try and make time to rest several times a day and ensure that you get adequate sleep by having early nights when possible. Have a warm bath with a few drops of jasmine, ylang ylang, or lavender oil to help relax the body ready for sleep. Yoga and swimming are perfect exercise for pregnancy and can energize you when you are feeling exhausted. They will also ensure a good night's sleep.

Early Night Bath Blend

During the times in pregnancy when you have less energy, add this calming concoction to a warm bath and try to get an early night as often as possible.

- 2 drops jasmine essential oil
- 2 drops lavender essential oil
- 2 drops ylang ylang essential oil

1. Mix ingredients together in a small bowl or amber jar.

2. Add to running bath water.

3. Sink in and enjoy for at least twenty minutes.

CHILDBIRTH

PRACTICING YOGA DURING PREGNANCY CAN HAVE AN AMAZING EFFECT ON THE body's ability to open to childbirth. Practicing the squat position is especially good for the pelvic region. An active birth, when you move around during childbirth and can give birth in an upright or all-fours position, rather than lying flat on your back, works with rather than against gravity.

When pregnant, it is a good idea to make up a natural birth toolkit to use during labor containing the natural remedies that can be used to ease the contractions and to help the body to heal afterwards. Below are some items you might like to include in your natural birth kit.

Natural Birth Toolkit

As you prepare for childbirth, it's important to include natural remedies on your list, such as essential oils and honey.

- A massage oil made with a few drops each of essential oils of clary sage and rose, added to 1½ fluid ounces (30 ml) base oil, such as organic sweet almond oil. Ask your midwife or partner to rub this into your lower back.

- Lavender and melissa essential oils, both of which can be applied to a handkerchief and inhaled to help you stay focused and used as a pick-me-up if you are feeling overwhelmed.

- Rescue Remedy, which can be taken for anxiety during labor and immediately after the birth to help the body begin the healing process. Add five drops to a glass of water and take small sips.

- A jar of honey to keep your strength up—a teaspoon can be taken as required.

- Red raspberry leaf tea can be drunk to help get labor started.

- Chamomile tea is useful in cases of anxiety or shaking.

Breastfeeding

A mother's milk is the perfect food for her baby. It contains all the essential nutrients and changes throughout development to provide exactly what the child needs at each stage. The first milk is called colostrum, a thick yellow milk that has high immune-boosting properties, especially important in the first days after the baby leaves the womb. The milk, which arrives around three days after birth, contains higher levels of proteins and fats to promote growth. A mother's milk continues to change to support the growing child and when a baby starts to eat solid food, the mother's breast milk adapts to provide more antibodies to protect the child's digestive system. In addition to the essential nutrients and immune-boosting properties that breastmilk offers, the act of breastfeeding is an important way to bond with a new baby. Skin-to-skin contact is vital for healthy development and breast feeding encourages production of the nurturing hormone, prolactin. There are natural remedies that you can take to increase milk flow and to help heal sore nipples.

If you can, it's a good idea to breastfeed your baby—this way they get essential nutrients and skin-to-skin contact.

As you prepare for childbirth, it's important to include natural remedies on your list, such as essential oils and honey.

Milk Production

The more a baby feeds, the more milk is produced, so an easy way to increase production is to feed your baby more frequently to get a good supply established. Fennel tea can also be taken to boost milk production.

Milk-Boosting Drink

- 1 ounce (25 g) fennel seeds
- 1 cup boiling water

1. Steep the fennel seeds in the boiling water.
2. Leave to infuse for ten minutes, strain, and then drink while still warm.
3. Take up to three times a day.

Sore, Cracked Nipples

A little expressed breastmilk massaged into the affected area can help to heal cracked nipples. This condition can be very painful but try to keep milk the flowing to prevent engorgement. If it is too uncomfortable to breastfeed on the affected breast, gently express milk by hand. Calendula salve can soothe sore skin and promotes healing. It is safe for babies to swallow.

Calendula Salve

- 2 ounces (50 g) beeswax
- 1 pan hot water
- 8 fluid ounces (250 ml) calendula oil (see page 91)
- A few drops rose essential oil

1. Melt the beeswax in a glass bowl over a pan of hot water.
2. Add the calendula oil and the rose essential oil.
3. Mix thoroughly and pour into a dark glass jar with a tight-fitting lid.
4. Store in the refrigerator and apply to sore nipples to help them heal.

Practice yoga during pregnancy, especially the squat position, to get your pelvic region prepared for childbirth.

Engorgement

During the first weeks after birth, your breasts can become full and hard. Feeding frequently should bring relief. Leaves from a Savoy cabbage kept cool in the refrigerator can be applied to the breasts to reduce swelling and absorb heat.

Your let-down reflex can be impacted by stress, so try to stay calm and relaxed when breastfeeding.

Problems With Let-Down

Breastfeeding is most effective when mother and baby are relaxed. If you are having problems relaxing, try having a warm bath with a few drops of lavender essential oil or make up a bottle of your own soothing milk flow bath oil. Try feeding your baby in the bath—you may find that the warm water helps them relax too.

Milk Flow Bath Oil

- 2 drops each of lavender, ylang ylang, and Roman chamomile essential oils
- 1½ fluid ounces (30 ml) organic sweet almond oil

1. Drop the essential oils into a glass jar and add the sweet almond oil.
2. Shake to mix and add a capful to warm water for a soothing bath.

Inflammation

Savoy cabbage leaves can be tucked inside your bra to calm inflammation. Echinacea tincture taken in a glass of water will help the body to fight infection. Calendula and chamomile essential oils are anti-inflammatory and can be diluted in a carrier oil, such as sweet almond, and massaged into your breasts.

Soothing Breast Oil

- 2 drops calendula essential oil
- 2 drops chamomile essential oil
- 1½ fluid ounces sweet almond oil

1. Drop the essential oils into a glass jar and add the sweet almond oil.
2. Shake to mix and gently massage into the breasts.

Fatigue

Rest when your baby is resting. Once breastfeeding is established you might find it comfortable to lie down on your side and rest whilst your baby is feeding. Ensure you are eating plenty of energy-rich foods and drinking lots of fluids to keep your energy levels up. Try slow-releasing energy foods such as oats, nuts, seeds, sprouts, and bananas.

It is natural to be tired as a new mother. Be sure to rest when your baby is resting and eat energy-rich foods.

MENOPAUSE

MENOPAUSE MARKS THE END OF MENSTRUATION, WHICH HAPPENS AT AROUND the age of fifty. There can be disorientating side effects such as hot flashes and memory loss. Clary sage is a great mood enhancer and balances the hormones. Place a few drops on to a handkerchief and inhale as required throughout the day. To reduce the incidence of night sweats, take a bath with chamomile essential oil before bed. Simply add a few drops to a warm bath.

Ensure that you get plenty of magnesium in the diet—nettles are a rich source and are available free on our doorsteps. Forget about expensive supplements and make yourself a nourishing nettle tonic. Don't worry about stings—the histamine is no longer active after the leaves have been boiled or blended.

Nettle Tonic

- Several handfuls nettle tops
- Boiling water, as needed

1. Place the nettle tops in a large saucepan. Cover with boiling water.
2. Boil for thirty minutes.
3. Strain through a muslin cloth and drink as required.

Menopause Tea

Motherwort is a traditional remedy for helping ease the body through this transition. Drink motherwort tea as often as needed.

- 1 ounce (25 g) dried motherwort
- 1 cup boiling water

1. Steep the dried motherwort in the boiling water.
2. Leave to infuse for ten minutes, strain, and drink while still warm.

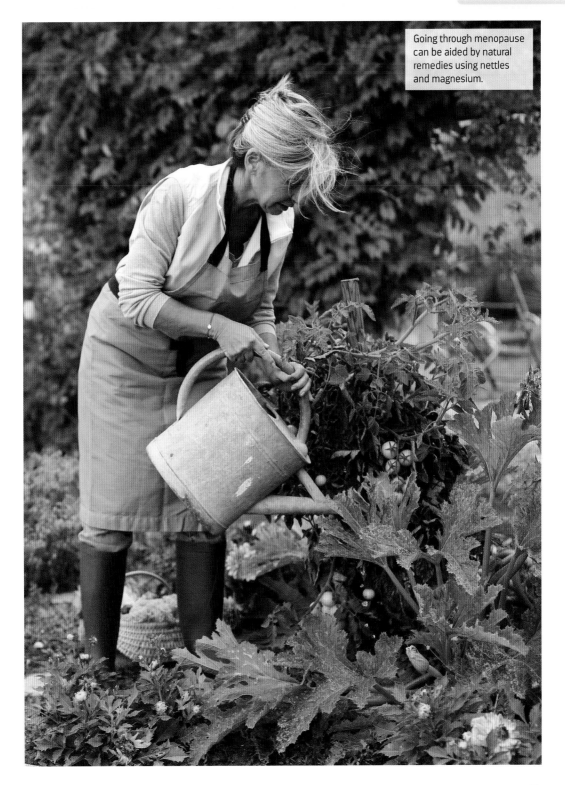

Going through menopause can be aided by natural remedies using nettles and magnesium.

Plant Profile: Motherwort

Motherwort has been an important herb since Roman times. The Latin name, *leonurus cardiaca*, is derived from the Greek word meaning "lion-hearted". The ancient Greeks used motherwort to relieve anxiety in mothers after childbirth. It really is a woman's herb, being valuable in the treatment of menstruation and menopausal problems as well as after childbirth. It is a member of the mint family, has a square stem, and opposite leaves. Small pink-and-lilac flowers appear on the upper part of the plant in summer. The plant grows to about a meter/yard in height and can be found along roadsides and in vacant fields and other waste areas.

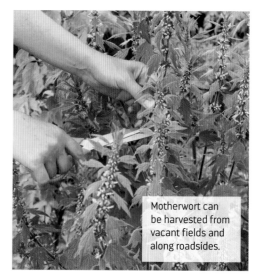

Motherwort can be harvested from vacant fields and along roadsides.

Today, motherwort is used to stimulate delayed or suppressed periods and to ease the discomfort of dysmenorrhea (painful menstruation). The plant contains constituents that act as a gentle uterine stimulant. It is for this reason that it should not be used in pregnancy, although after childbirth it helps to restore the uterus and to reduce the risk of bleeding after birth (postpartum hemorrhage).

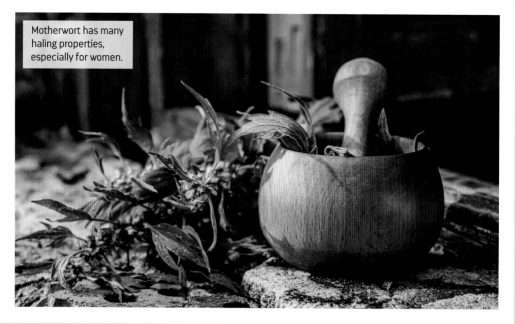

Motherwort has many haling properties, especially for women.

Take a motherwort tincture to ease your anxiety or when you need to calm your nerves.

Motherwort can be used during the menopausal years to treat hot flashes, fainting, stressed nerves, and sleep disorders. For hot flashes, add a few drops of tincture to a small glass of water and drink to harness the herb's great relaxing properties. Used regularly, motherwort feeds your nerves and your good common sense, relaxing and unclenching any held tension. Motherwort is not sedating but calming, leaving you ready for action, not flying off the handle or bouncing off the walls. Motherwort is your ally in tough times, and ten to twenty drops of tincture taken as soon as you feel your nerves starting to fray or just before a stressful event can have a wonderfully calming effect. This can be repeated every five minutes if needed.

Heart conditions are also treated with this common herb, *hence cardiaca* in the Latin name. It invigorates the circulation and increases oxygen in the blood. Motherwort calms a rapidly beating heart with readily usable minerals, trace elements, and an alkaloid exceptionally tonifying to the heart (and uterus). The German herbal doctor, Weiss, uses motherwort tincture for those with functional heart complaints. A dropperful of motherwort tincture acts quickly to ease palpitations and tachycardia (heartrate disorders). Regular use lowers hypertension, and sets you up to be a hale-hearted elder.

At night, motherwort's high calcium calming effect can be put to good use when you are awakened and have difficulty getting back to sleep. Keep a glass of water and a bottle of motherwort tincture by your bed and take ten to fifteen drops and a mouthful of water as soon as you wake.

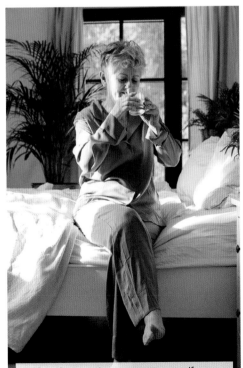

Add motherwort tincture to your water if you have difficulty getting back to sleep.

Plant Profile: Sweet Violet

Sweet violet (*viola odorata*) is an evergreen perennial. Although the plants are in leaf all year, it flowers from early spring. It is often found in areas of semi-shade such as woodland and grassy verges. In the kitchen, the leaves and flowers of sweet violet can be a welcome reminder of the warmer days to come. The flowers can be used as a colorful yet delicately flavored addition to a salad, or as a decoration for cakes and puddings.

Young leaves have a mild flavor, although they can become quite tough as they grow older. If you can find fresh, young leaves, they make a very good salad; their mild flavor enables them to be used in bulk.

Use sweet violet in salads, soups, teas, and more.

When added to soup they thicken in a similar way to okra. A soothing tea can be made from the leaves and flowers. For medicinal purposes, sweet violet has a long and proven history of folk use, especially in the treatment of cancer and whooping cough. It also contains salicylic acid, which is used to make aspirin. It is therefore effective in the treatment of headaches, migraines, and insomnia. The whole plant is anti-inflammatory, diaphoretic, diuretic, emollient, expectorant, and laxative. It is taken internally in the treatment of bronchitis, respiratory catarrh, coughs, asthma, and cancer of the breast, lungs, or digestive tract. Externally, it is used to treat mouth and throat infections.

Sweet violet flowers in early spring, but is in leaf all year.

The plant can either be used fresh, or harvested when it blooms and then dried for later use. The flowers are demulcent and emollient, and are used in the treatment of biliousness and lung troubles. The petals can be made into a syrup and used in the treatment of childhood illnesses, such as whooping cough. The roots are a much stronger expectorant than other parts of the plant, but they also contain the alkaloid violine, which at higher doses can be strongly purgative, causing diarrhea and vomiting. They are usually gathered in the autumn and dried for later use.

A homeopathic remedy is made from the whole fresh plant, which is considered useful in the treatment of spasmodic coughs and rheumatism of the wrist. An essential oil from the flowers is used in aromatherapy in the treatment of bronchial complaints, exhaustion, and skin complaints.

Plants can be grown as an effective weed-excluding ground cover when spaced about 11¾ inches (30 cm) apart. Sweet violet succeeds in most soils but prefers a cool, moist, well-drained humus-rich soil in partial or dappled shade and protection from winds. When grown in the open it prefers a moderately heavy rich soil. Sweet violets are very ornamental plants and there are many named varieties. They produce their delicately scented flowers in late winter and early spring—these are designed for fertilization by bees and since there are few bees around at this time of year, these flowers seldom set seed. However, the plants also produce a second type of flower later in the year. These never open, but seed is produced within them by self-fertilization. The plants will spread rapidly at the roots when they are growing well.

Most members of this genus have edible leaves and flower buds, although those species with yellow flowers can cause diarrhea if eaten in large quantities. Seed is best sown in the autumn in a cold frame. The seed requires a period of cold stratification, and the germination of stored seed can be erratic. Prick out the seedlings into individual pots when they are large enough to handle and plant them out in the summer. Divide in the autumn or just after flowering. Larger divisions can be planted out direct into their permanent positions. Plant out in the summer or the following spring.

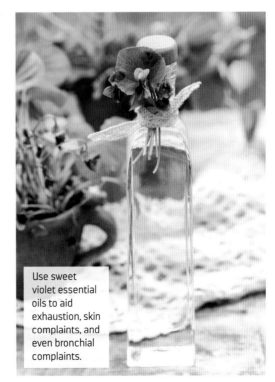

Use sweet violet essential oils to aid exhaustion, skin complaints, and even bronchial complaints.

BABIES AND CHILDREN

USING NATURAL MEDICINE IS A GENTLE AND REWARDING APPROACH TO YOUR family's health. Supporting and nurturing a child through an illness, whether it be a cold or chicken pox, can have a beneficial physiological effect on parent and child. Rather than resorting to pain-blocking over-the-counter drugs, treating the illness naturally aids the immune system and allows the body to fight the infection, making room for the developmental leap that often takes place after a period of convalescing.

In addition, holistic medicine treats the whole person rather than just the symptoms as in allopathic medicine. For example, a child with a cough and a sore throat is likely to be prescribed a cough suppressant and antibiotics by his doctor to treat their symptoms. A homeopath treating the same child will consult with the parent and, if appropriate, the child, to discover the child's general state of health and characteristics before providing a remedy that best treats the whole child—their mind, body, and soul.

Other holistic therapies work in the same way, treating the person, and not just the symptoms he or she is exhibiting. The most important advice when treating children is to listen to them. Children

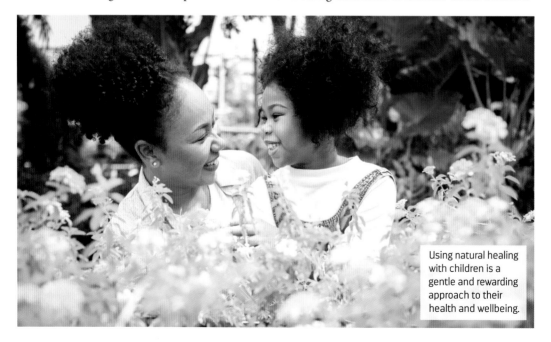

Using natural healing with children is a gentle and rewarding approach to their health and wellbeing.

have an amazing self-preservation instinct and often know exactly what they need to get better. Some children stop eating when they are ill, as their bodies need to concentrate on getting well rather than using precious energy to digest food. Other children crave specific foods or can tell you exactly what they need to feel better.

Sore Throat and Coughs

If your child has a sore throat, make some sage or thyme tea with honey.

Usually caused by an infection in the upper respiratory tract, a sore throat and cough can also be the symptoms of many other illnesses. Sage or thyme tea can be made with honey to soothe a sore throat. The homeopathic remedy Heper Sulph. can be used. Onions are a traditional remedy for soothing sore throats and easing coughs. Make your own cough medicine using the healing powers of honey and raw onion.

Coughing is nature's way of clearing an infection of the bronchial passages and protecting the lungs from damage. For this reason, do not suppress a cough. The homeopathic remedy Bryonia is effective at treating coughs and is available in piluled or syrup form. Echinacea boosts the immune system. A hot honey and lemon drink can be drunk as often as required. Place a teaspoon of honey and the juice of half a lemon in a cup, fill with boiling water, and allow to cool before drinking.

Cough Medicine

This makes an effective syrup for sore throats, coughs, and colds.

- ½ onion, cut into rings
- Honey, as needed

1. Place the onion into a shallow dish.

2. Cover with honey and leave to infuse overnight.

3. In the morning, strain and bottle the resulting liquid.

Colds

A cold is a natural purification process. If you discourage or suppress a cold, it could carry on in another form for many months. Get rest and drink plenty of fluids. Pulsatilla, the homeopathic remedy, is effective at treating colds with mucus. Ensure plenty of onions and garlic in the diet. A honey and lemon drink soothes and cleanses. A cup of ginger tea can be soothing and warming to the system.

Ginger Tea

- 1 small piece root ginger
- 1 cup boiling water
- 1 teaspoon honey, optional
- 1 teaspoon lemon juice, optional

1. Grate the root ginger into the boiling water.

2. Cover and leave for ten minutes.

3. Strain before serving and add the honey and lemon juice to boost the healing properties, if desired.

Croup

Croup is the acute inflammation and narrowing of the airways, which causes wheezing and whistling, breathing, and a barking cough. Spongia is the homeopathic remedy for croup. Steam inhalation can ease breathing.

Steam Inhaler

- 2 drops lavender or chamomile essential oil
- 1 large bowl boiling water

1. Place the essential oil in the bowl of boiling water.

2. Encourage your child to lean over and inhale the steam.

3. For babies and small children, take them into the bathroom and turn the shower on. The hot water will create the steam in the room, which will aid your child's breathing.

Chicken Pox

Chicken pox is a common viral infection, which causes a rash across the body—small red raised spots that develop into inflamed blisters—fever, and headache. Ensure plenty of rest and fluids. The homeopathic remedy Rhus Tox will soothe the skin irritation. Sponge the body with tepid water and add bicarbonate of soda to the bathwater to ease itching.

Earache

An earache is discomfort in the ear due to buildup of mucus. This can also be a symptom of mumps—if you suspect this is the case, see page 153 for advice. A hot water bottle placed over the ear can soothe the pain. Mullein oil, diluted in a carrier oil, can be dropped into the ear to ease discomfort.

Ear Drops

- 1 flowering spike of a mullein plant
- Organic sunflower oil, as needed
- 1½ fluid ounces (30 ml) sweet almond oil

1. Break the mullein plant into smaller pieces. Place in a pestle and add the sunflower oil.

2. Crush with the mortar to start releasing the beneficial parts of the plant.

3. Place in a large glass jar. Cover with more oil so that the plant is well covered, then put the lid on and shake well.

4. Leave outside in direct sunlight for twenty-one days.

5. Strain and pour in a dark bottle.

6. Add 1 teaspoon of this oil to the sweet almond oil. Use a pipette to apply three drops to each ear.

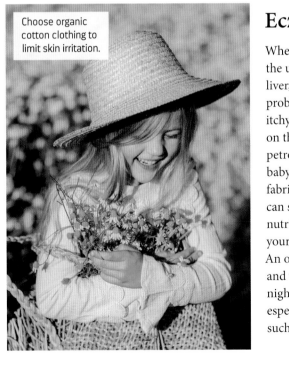

Choose organic cotton clothing to limit skin irritation.

Eczema

When the body cannot eliminate toxins through the usual channels, being the lungs, kidneys, or liver, the body expels them through the skin. Skin problems such as eczema are the result—a hot itchy rash that is usually found behind the knees, on the hands, feet, and behind the ears. Avoid petroleum-based products, soaps, and scented baby products and do not use detergents or fabric softeners to wash the family's clothes. Diet can sometimes be the cause. With the help of a nutritionist, try eliminating dairy products from your child's diet and the mother's if breastfeeding. An oat bath will soothe inflamed skin before bed and visualization can also be beneficial for a good night's sleep. Choose organic cotton clothing, especially for those items worn next to the skin, such as babygrows and underwear.

Instead of using chemical-based products to get rid of head lice, use an herbal treatment made of essential oils.

Head Lice

Head lice is an infestation of parasites that live one the scalp and in the hair. They can be very pervasive and tricky to get rid of. The most effective treatment is regularly brushing with a fine comb. Avoid the chemical-based products available in pharmacies, as these often contain powerful insecticides. Instead, use an herbal treatment to deter and remove head lice.

Herbal Head Lice Treatment

- 5 drops tea tree essential oil
- 5 drops eucalyptus essential oil
- 5 drops rosemary essential oil
- 5 drops lavender essential oil
- 3.4 fluid ounces (100 ml) sweet almond oil

1. Combine the essential oils with the sweet almond oil.

2. Rub into the child's hair and leave for twelve hours.

3. Wash out and comb thoroughly.

Measles

This is an infectious disease caused by a virus that begins like a cold, followed by a fever, which is accompanied by a rash. Flat brown-red spots usually come out on the ears and face. Lymph nodes will swell, and your child is likely to feel extremely unwell. Vomiting and diarrhea can also be symptoms. Ensure time for the child to rest and recuperate. Hot honey and lemon drinks are soothing and will help the body to heal. Add a few drops of lavender oil to cool water and sponge down. Also see fever on page 152.

Diaper Rash

A sore, itchy rash caused by wearing diapers. Refrain from using perfumed wipes, which can be a harsh irritant to delicate skin. Use a cotton flannel soaked in warm water instead. Allow plenty of diaper-free time, and apply calendula ointment to soothe sore skin.

Teething

The homeopathic remedies Chamomilla and Pulsatilla are recommended. Chamomile tea can also be helpful to ease the discomfort of new teeth coming through. Another method to help with teething pain is to use Baltic amber teething beads. These beads, often in the form of a necklace for your child, contain nontoxic Succinic acid. When worn against the skin, the beads warm up to the body temperature and release the helpful acid into the bloodstream. Succinic acid eases teething pain caused by inflammation and stimulates the thyroid gland to reduce drooling. Children can start wearing the beads from three months old to three years old. **These beads are not to be left with your child while they are sleeping or unattended. These beads are not to be chewed on, but rather worn against the skin.**

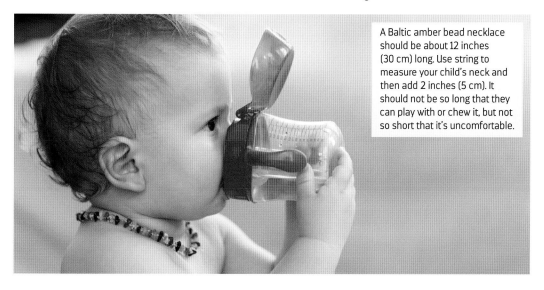

A Baltic amber bead necklace should be about 12 inches (30 cm) long. Use string to measure your child's neck and then add 2 inches (5 cm). It should not be so long that they can play with or chew it, but not so short that it's uncomfortable.

Fever

This is nature's most efficient healing tool. A fever is the body's mechanism for burning up unwanted matter to combat infection. A high temperature is to be encouraged as it is cleaning out the body. **However, it is vital to consult a doctor if your newborn baby is running a high temperature or if your child has ingested a poisonous substance**. A dry fever is dangerous, but a wet fever heals. Keep your child's fluid intake as high as possible—make sure that you have drinks that they like available. A rehydration drink can aid your child's recovery after diarrhea, vomiting, or during a fever. If breastfeeding, allow them to feed for as long and as often as they need.

If your child is refusing to drink, run a warm bath. Sponge with tepid water afterwards and dress your child in one thin cotton layer. Keep the environment well ventilated. Your child may choose not to eat during the fever, but this is perfectly normal. Encourage them to eat once the fever has passed.

Rehydration Drink

- 1 tablespoon sugar
- 1 tablespoon salt
- 18 fluid ounces (500 ml) filtered water
- 1¾ pint (1 liter) fresh apple juice

1. Place the sugar and salt in a jug.

2. Add the water and apple juice.

3. Encourage your child to drink throughout the day.

Mumps

This is a viral infection which causes fever and swelling of the lymph glands in the neck. Chamomile tea can be cooling and soothing to the system. Make a teapot of chamomile tea and pour a cup for your child. Allow the rest to cool, soak a cloth in the liquid, and then use to sponge and cool down the body. Cleavers (or sticky weed) is a cleansing herb for treating the mumps infection.

Cleaver Infusion

- 1 handful cleavers
- Boiling water, as needed

1. Gather the cleavers, chop them, and add to a cup. Cover with boiling water.
2. Leave to infuse for ten minutes.
3. Drink a cup a day while infection persists.

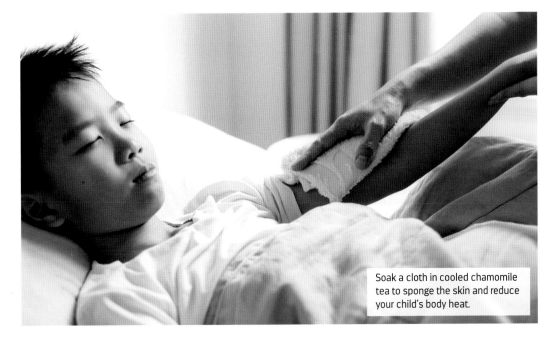

Soak a cloth in cooled chamomile tea to sponge the skin and reduce your child's body heat.

Plant Profile: Chamomile

Chamomile is one of nature's most healing and soothing plants, and has had a medicinal reputation in Europe for over 2,000 years. Plants have feathery green leaves and delicate daisylike flowers which, when crushed, give off a faint scent reminiscent of apples. It is this characteristic that led to the plant being called "ground-apple" by the Greeks—*kamai* meaning on the ground and *melon* meaning an apple. The Spanish call chamomile *manzanilla*, which translates as "a little apple," and give the same name to one of their lightest sherries, flavored with this plant.

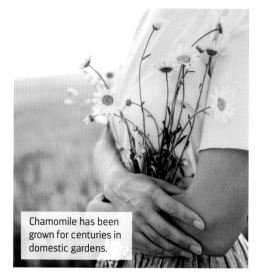
Chamomile has been grown for centuries in domestic gardens.

The Egyptians held this herb in the same high regard, and dedicated it to their gods because of its power to cure ague. It has been grown for centuries in domestic gardens, both as an excellent companion crop and for the many health benefits it offers. In the Middle Ages it was used as a strewing herb because of its lovely, pungent smell, and was planted in lawns as the scent is aroused through walking upon the plant. It has been called the "plant's physician" and some gardeners believe that if another plant is drooping or sickly it will recover if you place a chamomile plant near it. It is reputed to enhance the growth of cucumbers and onions if planted nearby.

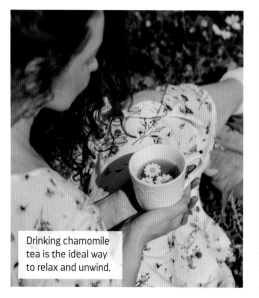
Drinking chamomile tea is the ideal way to relax and unwind.

Most are familiar with the refreshing taste of a cup of chamomile tea. An infusion of chamomile is an ideal way to relax and unwind. Studies have shown that the herb is an effective mild sedative and for this reason, is a great help in cases of insomnia. In cases of severe diarrhea, the soothing properties of chamomile come to the fore and an infusion can be sipped to ease painful stomachache and digestion. It relieves the vomiting caused by gastritis as well as heartburn. Chamomile is often used to help anorexia sufferers, as it improves the appetite. Herbalists have long relied upon chamomile as an herb to relieve menstrual cramps. Fresh and dried flowers in olive oil are used to treat painful joints and swellings. A cooled infusion makes a

Chamomile essential oil is useful to have around your home, and the flowers can be added to salads and desserts.

wonderful eye bath for tired and itchy eyes, which can prove invaluable for hay fever sufferers on days when the pollen count is high.

Camomile infusions are often used to bathe wounds and sores when the anti-inflammatory properties of the plant come into their own. These same properties make it a useful tea in cases of cystitis and kidney inflammation. It promotes the flow of urine and reduces fluid retention.

Rinsing your hair with an infusion of chamomile is a cheap and effective way of creating golden locks—this method was in practice long before peroxide was used to bleach the hair! Children have a particular affinity with chamomile, as it is so gentle and healing. Colic, teething pains, and infantile convulsions can all be aided. In a situation where a child is restless and fractious, cooled chamomile tea can have a positive soothing effect. It is also one of the most potent of cures for nightmares, in children and adults alike. It is used to dispel tension, fear, and emotional distress from the past, aiding emotional stability.

The essential oil of chamomile is a useful oil to have around the home. Chamomile essential oil is captured by steam distillation of the flower head and has a sweet, strong smell. In this form, it makes an excellent skincare oil and diluted in a carrier oil can be used in cases of acne, allergies, burns, eczema, dermatitis, psoriasis, and inflamed skin conditions. If you find yourself flying off the handle before your period, try massaging your abdomen with diluted chamomile essential oil to relax and comfort. Chamomile flowers can be added to salads and desserts; though the sweet smell masks a rather bitter taste, they make lovely decoration.

INDEX

acne, 84. *See also* boils
aconite, 16
addiction, 28
aloe vera, 13, 15, 17, 105, 131
anemia, 98
anemia, pregnancy, 127
angina, 98
Anti-Fungal Footbath, 85
anxiety, 29
Apple Cider Vinegar, 109
Apple Cider Vinegar Compress, 72
arnica, 14, 16, 105
arthritis, 108–9
asthma, 73

babies and children
  about: natural/holistic treatment for, 146–47; Rehydration Drink for, 152
  Chicken pox, 148
  croup, 148
  diaper rash, 151
  earache, 149
  eczema, 149
  fever, 152
  head lice, 150
  measles, 151
  sore throat and coughs, 147
  teething, 151
backache, 107–8, 127
Barley Water, 68
bath blends
  Comforting Ginger Root Footbath, 44
  Early Night Bath Blend, 133
  Epsom Salts Bath, 40
  Facial Steam Bath, 84
  Fear-Busting Bath Blend, 33
  Healing Steam Bath, 74
  Herbal Bath Bag, 31
  Milk Flow Bath Oil, 138
  Mustard Foot Bath, 75
  Oatmeal Bath, 81
  Peppermint Steam Bath, 71
  Relaxing Bath Blend, 32
  Stress-Away Bath Blend, 35
bites and stings, 15, 91
bladder inflammation (cystitis), 63
Bladder-Strengthening Tea, 63
bleeding gums, 128
blood pressure, 97
body scan meditation, 9–10

boils, 89
bones, muscles, and joints
  about: comfrey profile for, 110–11; treating and maintaining good health, 103–4
  arthritis, 108–9
  backache, 107–8, 127
  fractures, 105
  osteoporosis, 104
  rheumatism, 106
  sprains and pulled muscles, 105
borage, growing and uses, 22–23
Borage Tincture, 30
breastfeeding, 120, 135–36
broken bones, 105
bronchitis/lung infection, 74
burns and scalds, 17. *See also* sunburn

Cabbage Poultice, 86
calendula
  Calendula Extract, 116
  Calendula Oil, 91
  Calendula Salve, 136
  growing, 20–21, 93
  plant profile, 92–93
  uses/qualities, 14, 20–21, 92–93
Carrot Juice, 53
catarrh, 75
Cayenne Oil, 106
celery seed, for flatulence, 54
Celery Seed Tonic, 62
chamomile
  Chamomile, Fennel, and Thyme Infusion, 132
  Chamomile Massage Oil, 81
  Chamomile Tea, 32
  growing, 22
  plant profile, 154–55
  uses/qualities, 14, 16, 17, 22, 55, 154–55
Chicken pox, 148
Chickweed Infusion, 115
chilblains, 85
childbirth
  about: natural birth toolkit, 134; yoga and, 133, 134, 137
  breastfeeding, 120, 135–36
  engorgement, 137
  let-down problems, 138

milk production, 136, 138
  sore, cracked nipples, 136
children. *See* babies and children
Cleansing Tonic, 17
Cleaver Infusion, 153
cloves, 14
cold sores, 87
colds, 70, 148
Comforting Ginger Root Footbath, 44
comfrey
  Comfrey Oil, 109
  Comfrey Ointment, 16, 84
  Comfrey Tea, 104
  plant profile, 110–11
  uses/qualities, 14, 110–11
common cold, 70, 148
compresses
  Apple Cider Vinegar Compress, 72
  Compress for Migraine Attacks, 43
  Cool Compress for Sunburn, 78
  Hot Compress for Period Pains, 77
  Pilewort Compress, 99
  Witch Hazel Compress, 100
conjunctivitis, 114
constipation, 52, 128
Cool Compress for Sunburn, 78
Cooling Tea, 87
Cough Medicine, 147
coughs, 73, 147. *See also* common cold
cramps, during pregnancy, 129
Crohn's disease, 55
croup, 148
cuts and wounds/sores, 16, 86
cystitis, 28, 63, 155

dandelion, 56–58
dandruff, 90
Decongestant Temple Rub, 75
deodorant recipes, 83
depression, 30
diaper rash, 151
diarrhea, 53
digestive system. *See also* engorgement, childbirth and
  about: diet, eating habits and, 48–49; guidelines

for treating/maintaining, 48–50; liver and liver problems, 49–50; milk thistle and, 54, 59–60; stomach acid, 49; ulcers and "Stomach fire," 49
constipation, 52, 128
Crohn's disease, 55
diarrhea, 53
flatulence, 54
hepatitis, 54
indigestion and heartburn, 52, 129
irritable bowel syndrome (IBS), 53
nausea and vomiting, 50
stomachache, 51
travel sickness, 51
Dill Infusion, 52
dizziness, 97, 127, 130

Ear Drops, 149. *See also* eyes and ears
Early Night Bath Blend, 133
eczema, 81, 149
Elderflower Nasal Wash, 71
Elderflower Tea, 69
emotions. *See* mind and emotions
Energy-Boosting Dandelion Tea, 57
engorgement, childbirth and, 137
epilepsy, 45
Epsom Salts Bath, 40
exercise, mental health and, 27
eyebright (*Euphrasia officinalis*), about, 112–13
Eyebright Infusion, 114
eyes and ears
  about: fennel plant profile and, 118–20; overview of remedies for, 112–13
  conjunctivitis, 114
  ear wax buildup, 116
  earache, 149
  eyestrain, 115
  middle ear infection, 117
  Soothing Eye Bath, 38, 114
  styes, 116

Facial Steam Bath, 84
fatigue, pregnancy/childbirth, 133, 139

Fear Diffuser, 33
Fear-Busting Bath Blend, 33
fennel
    Chamomile, Fennel, and
        Thyme Infusion, 132
    Fennel Tea, 129
    plant profile, 118–20
fertility, 125
fever, 152
first aid kit, herbal, 15–17
flatulence, 54
flu, 68
fluid retention, 130
food poisoning, 17
footbaths, 44, 75, 85
fractures, 105

garlic
    Garlic Syrup, 74
    Garlic Tincture, 73
    growing, 24
    uses/qualities, 13, 24
gas (flatulence), 54
ginger
    Comforting Ginger Root
        Footbath, 44
    uses/qualities, 14
    Warming Ginger Tea, 50
Growing Bump Oil, 131
growing herbs/medicine, 18–24.
    See also specific herbs
gums, bleeding, 128

hair
    dandruff, 90
    losing, 89
hawthorn
    Hawthorn Berry Brandy, 97
    Hawthorn Infusion, 98
    plant profile, 101–2
hay fever, 69
head lice, 150
headache, 44. See also migraine
Healing Skin Lotion, 88
Healing Steam Bath, 74
hearing. See eyes and ears
heart and blood health
    about: diet and, 96; hawthorn
        plant profile and, 101–2;
        importance of, 95–96; men
        and, 94–95; motherwort
        and, 98, 143 (See also
        Nurturing Tea); nourishing
        the heart, 95
    anemia, 98
    angina, 98
    hemorrhoids, 99, 131 (See
        also Witch Hazel Compress)
    high blood pressure, 97
    low blood pressure, 97
    varicose veins, 100
heartburn and indigestion,
    52, 129
hemorrhoids, 99, 131. See also
    Witch Hazel Compress
hepatitis, 54

Herbal Bath Bag, 31
herbal first aid kit, 15–17
Herbal Head Lice Treatment,
    150
herbs. See plants/herbs
high blood pressure, 97
honey, uses/qualities, 14, 17
Honey and Onion Syrup, 70
Horseradish Poultice, 85
Hot Compress for Period
    Pains, 77
hypericum, 16

IBS, 53
ignatia, 16
incontinence, stress, 63
indigestion and heartburn,
    52, 129
infusions, decoctions, and
    tonics
    Celery Seed Tonic, 62
    Chamomile, Fennel, and
        Thyme Infusion, 132
    Chickweed Infusion, 115
    Cleansing Tonic, 17
    Dill Infusion, 52
    Eyebright Infusion, 114
    Hawthorn Infusion, 98
    Licorice Infusion, 52
    Nettle Tonic, 140
    Peppermint Infusion, 55
    Rose Petal Infusion, 115
    Yarrow Infusion, 117
inhaler, steam, 148
insect bites, 15, 91
insomnia, 31, 130, 143
irritable bowel syndrome
    (IBS), 53

joints. See bones, muscles, and
    joints
juice, carrot, 53
juice, lemon, 53

kidney stones, 62
kits
    essential home remedy kit,
        13–14
    herbal first aid kit, 15–17
    natural birth toolkit, 134
    portable, items to include, 15,
        16, 17

lavender
    Cool Compress for Sunburn,
        78
    growing, 21, 78
    Hot Compress for Period
        Pains, 77
    oil uses/qualities, 14, 15, 16,
        17, 21, 76–78
    plant profile, 76–78
lemon balm, 24. See also
    Nurturing Tea
lemon juice, 13
lice, head, 150

Licorice Infusion, 52
liniment, seaweed, 106
Liquid Deodorant, 83
liver and liver problems, 49–50,
    54, 57. See also digestive
    system; milk thistle
Liver Tonic Dandelion
    Decoction, 57
lotion, healing skin, 88
Love Your Liver Tincture, 54
Lovers' Massage Oil, 37
low blood pressure, 97
lung infection/bronchitis, 74.
    See also respiratory system

massage
    blood pressure and, 97
    Chamomile Massage Oil, 81
    cramps and, 129
    de-stress tip, 36
    fluid retention and, 130
    Lovers' Massage Oil, 37
    Massage Oil for Sprains, 105
    Massage Oil for Varicose
        Veins, 100
    Moontime Massage Oil, 124
    multiple sclerosis, and 40
    natural birth oil recipe, 134
    oil for backache, 107
    pelvic pain and, 131
    for prickly heat, 82
    Soothing Massage Oil, 127
measles, 151
meditation, benefits of, 27, 59
meditation, body scan, 9
memory loss, 29
menopause, 140–41. See also
    motherwort
Menopause Tea, 140
menstrual cycle, 77, 123–24.
    See also Hot Compress for
    Period Pains
middle ear infection, 117
migraine, 43
milk production
    about, 136
    Milk Flow Bath Oil, 138
    Milk-Boosting Drink, 138
milk thistle, 54, 59–60
mind and emotions. See also
    stress
    about: guidelines for treating,
        26–27
    addiction, 28
    anxiety, 29
    depression, 30
    insomnia, 31, 130
    memory loss, 29
    obsessive-compulsive disorder
        (OCD), 32
    phobias, 33
Moontime Massage Oil, 124
morning sickness, 130
motherwort, 98, 142–43. See
    also Nurturing Tea
Mullein Oil, 117

multiple sclerosis, 39–40
muscles. See bones, muscles,
    and joints
Mustard Footbath, 75
Mustard Poultice, 108

nasal wash, elderflower, 71
natural home remedies
    about: author's background,
        8–9; using this book and,
        10, 11
    body scan meditation and,
        9–10
    essential home remedy kit,
        13–14
    herbal first aid kit, 15–17
    plant knowledge and, 12
    self-awareness and, 9
nausea and vomiting, 50
Nerve Tonic, 41
nervous system. See also stress
    epilepsy, 45
    headache, 44
    migraine, 43
    multiple sclerosis, 39–40
    neuralgia, 46
    Parkinson's disease, 41
    shingles, 42
    stroke, 41
nettles
    Nettle Tea, 98
    Nettle Tonic, 140
    plant profile, 65–66
neuralgia, 46
nipples, sore/cracked, 136
nosebleeds, 72
Nurturing Tea, 29

Oat Water, 28
Oatmeal Bath, 81
obsessive-compulsive disorder
    (OCD), 32
oils
    Calendula Oil, 91
    Cayenne Oil, 106
    Chamomile Massage Oil, 81
    Comfrey Oil, 109
    Growing Bump Oil, 131
    Lovers' Massage Oil, 37
    Massage Oil for Sprains, 105
    Massage Oil for Varicose
        Veins, 100
    Milk Flow Bath Oil, 138
    Moontime Massage Oil, 124
    Mullein Oil, 117
    Plantain Oil, 91
    Soothing Massage Oil, 127
osteoporosis, 104

Parkinson's disease, 41
pelvic pain, 131
peppermint
    Cooling Tea, 87
    Peppermint Infusion, 55
    Peppermint Steam Bath, 71
    uses/qualities, 14

perspiration, 83
phobias, 33
Pilewort Compress, 99
plant profiles
calendula, 92–93
chamomile, 154–55
comfrey, 110–11
dandelion, 56–58
fennel, 118–20
hawthorn, 101–2
lavender, 76–78
milk thistle, 59–60
motherwort, 142–43
nettle, 65–66
rose, 37–38
rosemary, 46–47
sweet violet, 144–45
plantain
Plantain Oil, 91
Plantain Tincture, 42
uses/qualities, 15
plants/herbs. See also specific
plants/herbs
growing, 18–24
herb spiral, 18–24
knowledge of, 12
pneumonia, 73–74
poultices
Cabbage Poultice, 86
Horseradish Poultice, 85
Mustard Poultice, 108
pregnancy
about: milk thistle and, 60;
natural remedies and herbs
to avoid, 126; yoga and,
127, 129
anemia, 127
backache, 127
bleeding gums, 128
constipation, 128
cramps, 129
dizziness, 130
fluid retention, 130
hemorrhoids, 131
indigestion, 129
insomnia, 130
morning sickness, 130
pelvic pain, 131
stretch marks, 131
thrush, 132
tiredness, 133
prickly heat, 82
psoriasis, 82
pulled muscles and sprains, 105

Quick-Healing Tea, 70

rashes, 88
Rehydration Drink, 152
Relaxing Bath Blend, 32
rescue remedy, about, 14, 15,
16, 17
respiratory system
about: lavender for, 76–78
(See also lavender); nasal

wash for, 71; problems and
remedies, 67
asthma, 73
catarrh, 75
common cold, 70, 148
coughs, 73, 147
croup, 148
flu, 68
hay fever, 69
lung infection/bronchitis, 74
nosebleeds, 72
pneumonia, 73–74
sinusitis, 71
sore throat, 72
rheumatism, 106
Rose Petal Infusion, 115
rose plant profile, 37–38
rosehip tea, energy-boosting, 51
rosemary
essential oil, 47
growing and uses, 21, 46–47
plant profile, 46–47
Rosemary Tea, 29, 41

Sage Tea, 89
scalds and burns, 17
Seaweed Liniment, 106
shingles, 42
shock, mild, 16
sight. See eyes and ears
sinusitis, 71
skin. See also sunburn
about: indicating imbalances
throughout the body,
79–80; as largest organ, 79
acne, 84
athlete's foot, 85
boils, 89
chilblains, 85
cold sores, 87
cuts and sores, 86
dandruff, 90
eczema, 81, 149
hair loss, 89
insect bites, 91
Oatmeal Bath, 81
perspiration, 83
prickly heat, 82
psoriasis, 82
rashes, 88
sunstroke, 17, 87
warts, 88
sleep, insomnia treatments, 31,
130, 143
Soothing Eye Bath, 38, 114
Soothing Massage Oil, 127
Soothing Nettle Tea, 66
sore throat, 72
sorrel, 24
sprains and pulled muscles, 105
St. John's Wort Oil, 46
St. John's Wort Tincture, 87
steam baths, 71, 74, 84
Steam Inhaler, 148
stings and bites, 15, 91

stomach acid, 49. See also
digestive system
stomachache, 51
strawberry, wild, 23
stress, 34–36. See also nervous
system
acknowledging, 34–35
chamomile oil and, 155
de-stress tips, 35
impact/effects of, 34, 39
natural remedies, 35
Stress-Away Bath Blend, 35
stress incontinence, 63
stretch marks, 131
stroke, 41
styes, 116
sunburn
about: treating, 90–91
Calendula Oil, 91
Cool Compress for Sunburn,
78
sunstroke, 17, 87
sweet violet, 24, 144–45
syrup
Cough Medicine, 147
Garlic Syrup, 74
Honey and Onion Syrup, 70

tea. See also infusions,
decoctions, and tonics
about: calming stress, 34
Bladder-Strengthening
Tea, 63
Chamomile Tea, 32
Comfrey Tea, 104
Cooling Tea, 87
Elderflower Tea, 69
Energy-Boosting Dandelion
Tea, 57
Fennel Tea, 129
Menopause Tea, 140
Nettle Tea, 98
Nurturing Tea, 29
Quick-Healing Tea, 70
Red Raspberry Tea, 128
Sage Tea, 89
Soothing Nettle Tea, 66
Vital Energy-Boosting
Rosehip Tea, 51
Warming Ginger Tea, 50
Yarrow or Rosemary Tea, 41
tea tree oil, about, 16
teething, 151
throat, sore, 72
thrush, 132
thyme, 89, 132, 147
tinctures
Garlic Tincture, 73
Love Your Liver Tincture, 54
St. John's Wort Tincture, 87
Yarrow Tincture, 86
tiredness, pregnancy/childbirth,
133, 139
tonics. See infusions, decoctions,
and tonics

travel sickness, 51
treatment uses/qualities
Rosemary Tea, 29

urinary system
about: kidney imbalance, 62;
water/nutrition guidelines
for health of, 61–62
cystitis, 28, 63, 155
kidney stones, 62
stress incontinence, 63
urinary complaints, 63
urine therapy, 64

varicose veins, 100
vinegar
Apple Cider Vinegar, 109
Apple Cider Vinegar
Compress, 72
Rosemary Vinegar, 90
vision. See eyes and ears
Vital Energy-Boosting Rosehip
Tea, 51
vomiting and nausea, 50

Warming Ginger Tea, 50
warts, 88
water, barley, 68
wild strawberry, 23
Witch Hazel Compress, 100
women's health. See also babies
and children; childbirth;
pregnancy
about: overview of, 121–22
fertility, 123–24
menopause, 140–41 (See also
motherwort)
menstrual cycle, 77, 123–24
(See also Hot Compress for
Period Pains)
wounds and cut, 16

Yarrow Infusion, 117
Yarrow or Rosemary Tea, 41
Yarrow Tincture, 86
yoga
aiding sleep, 31
childbirth and, 133, 134, 137
eye fatigue and, 113
hair growth and, 89
multiple sclerosis and, 39, 40
pregnancy and, 127, 129
relieving tension and
blockages, 10, 107
Yoga Nidra, 31

Photo Credits

All images are from Shutterstock.com

GoodStudio (illustrations on footers and pages 1, 9, 22, 25, 35, 37, 39, 41 top, 47, 51, 61, 67, 79, 107, 120–21, 125, 134, and 160), marilyn barbone (2; 30, middle; 54); Sea Wave (4–5, 29, bottom); Dragon Images (6; 44, top; 55, top); Nataly Studio (8); Boyki.Pictures (8); Mariia Korneeva (9, top); A.Azarnikova (10, top; 126, bottom); Alena_Kos (10, bottom); Snowbelle (11); Marina_Popmarleo (11, 26); theshots.co (12, top); Natalia Lisovskaya (12, bottom); Mahony (13); Foxyliam (herb illustrations on pages 13–14, 24, 29, 33, 41 bottom–42, 51–54, 62, 71–73, 75, 82, 85, 87, 104, 106, 116, 128, 130, 136, 139–140, 151, 153); MAXSHOT.PL (15, top); Vasilyeva Ekaterin (15, bottom); Yanya (16, middle); Madeleine Steinbach (16, bottom; 45, middle; 63, bottom; 66; 80, bottom; 84, middle; 110, bottom; 111; 124, top); CreatoraLab (17, middle top); Pixel-Shot (17, middle bottom; 78, top; 105, bottom; 136, top); encierro (18, 113); terra incognita (19); Joshua Resnick (20, top); 1777177 (20, bottom; 142, top); Anna Odessitka (21, top); Caterina Trimarchi (21, bottom); Mariana Romaniv (22); FotoHelin (23, top; 35; 42, top; 75, bottom); nnattalli (23, bottom; 59, bottom); Kris Jacques (24); Dmytro Zinkevych (25); Iryna Inshyna (26; 80, top; 154, top); Jlco Julia Amaral (27); Katrin Friedl Fotografie (28, top); FamStudio (28, bottom); Georgina198 (29, middle); Michael Kraus (30, bottom); RealPeopleStudio (31, top); kosmos111 (31, bottom); Vera Prokhorova (32, top); Valentyn Volkov (32, middle); Nikolay Litov (32, bottom); DinaSova (33, middle); New Africa (33, bottom; 63, middle; 71, bottom; 81, middle; 83, middle; 84, bottom; 91, bottom; 121; 130); Alena Ozerova (34); LizavetaS (34, illustration); Marish (35 illustrations); oksana2010 (37, top); Maryna Pleshkun (37, bottom); Olga Miltsova (38, top); eva_blanco (38, bottom); maruco (38, bottom); ShaikhMeraj (40, top); elizabethmphl (40, bottom); Tatiana_Pink (41, middle); Heike Rau (41, bottom; 147, bottom); Auhustsinovich (42, bottom); Elena Elisseeva (43, middle; 89, top); NDAB Creativity (43, bottom; 95); puhhha (44, bottom); inewsfoto (45, bottom); Alena Yudina (46); Esin Deniz (46, 118); Microgen (47); Art_Photo (48); Prisca Laguna (49, top); Tatevosian Yana (49, bottom); pilipphoto (50, top); gpointstudio (50, bottom); Sunvic (51); Oksana Shufrych (52, middle); Luis Echeverri Urrea (52, bottom); Beliphotos (53, middle); Beatriz Vera (53, bottom); chakad (55, bottom); Diana Taliun (56); mentalmind (56, 115); shurkin_son (57, top); Tati Liberta (57, bottom; 129, bottom); OleynykO (58); Soyka (59, top); Just Life (60); Kostikova Natalia (61); ideyweb (62, top); Serena Carminati (62); Edalin Photography (63, top); Lunov Mykola (65, top; 85, bottom; 88, middle); Slatan (65, bottom); Mix and Match Studio (67); Africa Studio (68, top); Igogosha (68, 73); Indian Food Images (68, bottom); JPC-PROD (69, top); Lipatova Maryna (69, bottom; 142, bottom; 149, top; 153, top); pizzastereo (70); juliaap (70, middle); Mariya Surmacheva (70, bottom); Antonova Ganna (71, middle); Ermolaev Alexander (72, top); 279photo Studio (72, bottom); Maryna Osadcha (73, 116); Pat_Hastings (74, top); Kinek00 (74, bottom); plprod (75, middle); Marina Bakush (76); Olga in Helsinki (77); sukiyaki (77); Iarisa Stefanjuk (78); BLACKDAY (79); Dmytro Zinkevuch (81, top); Milenie (81, bottom); BearFotos (82); Prostock-studio (83, bottom; 97; 139); metamorworks (84, top); YueStock (85, middle); Sokor Space (85, bottom); Helen Sushitskaya (86, top); NatalyaBond (87, top); Jeronimo Vilaplana (87, bottom); Shidlovski (88, top); KieferPix (88, bottom); Anastassiya Bezhekeneva (89, middle); amberto4ka (89, bottom); Fernanda_Reyes (90, top); triocean (90, middle); Siberian Art (90); Khomulo Anna (91, top); lemono (91, 92); Maria Aleshina (92); Alis Photo (93); Glinskaja Olga (91); TimeImage Production (91); Nungning20 (97, top); LN team (97, middle; 98, top; 155); Tani Kuzminka (97, bottom); Rawpixel.com (98, middle); Strela Studio (98, bottom); Elena Khus (99); shansh23 (99); Albina Gavrilovic (100, top); Tatjana Baibakova (100, middle); Maren Winter (100, bottom); Xiangli Li (101, top); Try_my_best (101, bottom); Bogdan Sonjachnyj (102, top); teatian (102, bottom); Irina Gorbunovair (103); fizkes (103; 104, top); Cloud Cap Photography (104, bottom); Yurii_Yarema (105, top); Tijana Simic (105, middle); kazmulka (106, middle); Manfred Ruckszio (106, bottom); AnnaStills (107); FotosDo (108, top); Pressmaster (108, bottom); zetat (109, top); VICUSCHKA (109, middle); Natspace (109); Marina Lohrbach (110, top); Miroslav Hlavko (112, top); Monkey Business Images (112, bottom); Natty_Blissful (114); Mikhail Kadochnikov (114, middle); beta7 (114, bottom); Gulnazina Javda (115, middle); ElenVik (115, bottom); Akemaster (117, top); badnews86dups (117, middle); VIRTEXIE (117, bottom); VH-studio (119); AmyLv (120); CCISUL (121); Dean Drobot (122); PCH.Vector (123); ViDI Studio (124, bottom); Krakenimages.com (125, right); Kerkdanno (125, left); Alla_vector (126); Marta Nogueira (126, top); Jacob Lund (127, top); Botamochy (127, bottom); Y.P.photo (128); Josep Suria (129, top); Bowonpat Sakaew (131, middle); Gee363 (131, bottom); Baba.Images (132, top); irina02 (132, bottom); Helga Khorimarko (133); Racamani (133); Irina Qiwi (134); Nastyaofly (135, middle); comzeal images (135, bottom); rawf8 (136, bottom); Taras Grebinets (137); Alina.Alina (137); SeventyFour (138, top); Deazer (138, bottom); Tatiana Belova (139, top); Albina Bugarcheva (140); goodluz (141); 13Smile (143, top); Ground Picture (143, bottom); Magdanatka (144, top); Olga_Shestakova (144, bottom); Agnes Kantaruk (145); Visual Generation (146); Manop Boonpeng (146); JeannieR (147, top); Halfpoint (148, top); Teresa Kasprzycka (148, bottom); Maples Images (149, bottom); riopatuca (150, top); photopixel (150, bottom); anastasia.gis (151); Petar Djordjevic (151); marcin jucha (152); The img (152); TinnaPong (153, bottom); Olga Savina (154, bottom).

About the Author

Melissa Corkhill has long been making herbal remedies for family and friends. She trained in naturopathy after the birth of her first child and has gone on to study yoga and nutrition, shamanism, and cycle awareness. She has also undertaken work as an herbal apprentice to a medical herbalist and founded a magazine about environmental issues and natural living twenty years ago.

Raised by a pioneering spirit interested in natural medicine, Melissa is lucky to have been given a grounding in the mystery and wonder of nature from a very early age by her mother.

The magazine she founded, *The Green Parent* is still going strong today and is packed with information about choosing an alternative lifestyle, including foraging for, and making, your own medicines from the plants that grow around you.

Passionate about the healing power of plants, Melissa can usually be found in her wild garden on the south coast of England, or walking the chalk downland near where she lives with a foraging bag packed with berries, leaves, and nuts.

She is often accompanied by the youngest of her three children, all of whom have been brought up to make their own balms and salves from nature's medicine chest.

Melissa is excited that this book will help you on the road to a deeper relationship with nature. She believes that this innate connection to the plants around us is vital to the survival of our planet and the source of greater wellbeing for all of us.